$4.95

OTHER VOLUMES IN
EXERCISES IN DIAGNOSTIC RADIOLOGY

EXERCISES IN DIAGNOSTIC RADIOLOGY

3

BONE

LUCY FRANK SQUIRE, M.D.

Lecturer, Harvard Medical School; Visiting Radiologist,
Massachusetts General Hospital, Boston, Massachusetts;
Associate Professor of Radiology, State University of
New York, Downstate Medical Center, Brooklyn, N.Y.

WILLIAM M. COLAIACE, M.D.

Clinical Instructor in Radiology, Tufts University
School of Medicine; Clinical Instructor, Brown University;
Radiologist, Roger Williams General Hospital,
Providence, Rhode Island

NATALIE STRUTYNSKY, M.D.

Assistant Professor, Radiology, New York Medical College,
New York City

W. B. SAUNDERS COMPANY • PHILADELPHIA • LONDON • TORONTO

W. B. Saunders Company: West Washington Square
                           Philadelphia, PA.   19105

                           12 Dyott Street
                           London, WC1A   1DB

                           833 Oxford Street
                           Toronto, Ontario M8Z 5T9, Canada

Exercises in Diagnostic Radiology—Volume 3   Bone   ISBN 0-7216-8527-7

Print No.:   9   8   7   6   5   4

PREFACE FOR STUDENTS AND TEACHERS

In the past several years there has been a gratifying reassessment of the place of radiology in the curricula of medical schools. The result has been that there are now fewer students leaving medical school without some introduction to the use of radiologic methods in the clinical study of the chest and abdomen. The increasing use of special radiographic procedures, of ever greater delicacy of execution, has begun to lend to the specialty some of the glamour formerly reserved for the cardiac or neurological surgeon.

In the midst of all this, application of the roentgen method to the study of *bone* has become the private reserve of the orthopedist and the practicing radiologist, in spite of the fact that it was probably the very first practical medical application and apparent to Roentgen himself. The student is often left with only a sketchy idea of what bones look like radiographically and, worse, little knowledge of the important part bone plays in the economy of the human organism, or of the extent to which the radiographic study documents changes in that economy.

This volume is an attempt to place the radiologic study of bone upon the same logical foundation as that of the chest and abdomen—for the medical student. It follows that this workbook is somewhat more didactic than the first two, particularly on the subject of bone growth. We have continued to use the problem-answer format, however, and are encouraged to do so by the favorable response of both students and teachers to this approach.

We do not wish to offer the usual demurrers for omissions or superficial treatment of certain subjects but would remind the reader that the book is not intended to be even an abbreviated survey of the roentgen manifestations of bone disease. The material has been chosen solely on the strength of the principle illustrated, with little regard for the rarity of some of the diseases presented.

We urge the student to reread Chapter 16 in *Fundamentals of Roentgenology* (L.F.S.) as an introduction to the material presented here.

WILLIAM M. COLAIACE

Roger Williams General Hospital
825 Chalkstone Avenue
Providence, R. I. 02908

ACKNOWLEDGMENTS

If it had not been for the generosity of Drs. Jack Edeiken and Philip Hodes of the Jefferson Medical College, the writing of this volume might have been delayed far into the future. Their loan of illustrations from *Roentgenologic Diagnosis of Diseases of Bone*, 1967, provided the nucleus of material around which the book took form. Thanks are also due to their publisher, The Williams & Wilkins Company, for agreeing to our re-use of the material.

We have also to thank the Harvard University Press, The Commonwealth Fund, and our friends at the Eastman Kodak Company for the use and re-use of materials originally collected for *Fundamentals of Roentgenology* (L.F.S.).

We are especially indebted to Dr. Deborah Forrester for a meticulous examination of the manuscript and some excellent critical ideas.

We would not allow the manuscript to appear in print without the prior approval of members of its intended audience. Four medical students, Howard Marcus (Tufts University), Robert F. Stephens (Washington University, St. Louis, Mo.), Elbert H. Magoon (Harvard University), and Steele Belok (New York University School of Medicine) gave up two evenings of their valuable time to keep us on the tracks of clarity and accuracy. We owe them our special thanks.

Roy Wall, Medical Illustrator for the Roger Williams General Hospital in Providence, R. I.; Francis de L. Cunningham of New York City; and Edith Tagren of the Department of Medical Illustration at the Massachusetts General Hospital prepared the drawings and diagrams. Their work is much appreciated.

Mrs. Marion Leigh typed much of the manuscript and arranged the index. Her accuracy and efficiency are greatly appreciated.

Lastly, we wish to thank the many students whose pleas for a short introduction to the radiology of bone convinced us of the need for such a book. We hope—and expect—that if we have succeeded in our aim, the students will go on to the many excellent larger works available on the subject.

L. F. S.

W. M. C.

N. S.

INTRODUCTION

It may now be difficult for you to recall your bewilderment when first confronted with radiographs of the chest and abdomen. The apparently endless variety of shape, size, density, and lucency has by this time yielded to systematic analysis, sharpened powers of observation, and, surely, increased knowledge of anatomy and physiology. Doubts may return when you face the fact that, though an individual has but one chest and one abdomen, he has 206 bones (more or less), all of them different in size, shape, and function. Generations of unfortunate medical students have spent many hours committing to memory all the protuberances, ridges, notches, and processes of bone.

Let us celebrate together the declining popularity of such activity, and proceed to a consideration of what bones really are — a uniform organ system with intricate structural and functional connections with all other organ systems in the body.

In correlating roentgen changes in bone with pathology, you will be happy to know that what you see in radiographs of bones indicates much more definitely what the histopathologic change is likely to be than in the chest and abdomen. For example, you will remember that there were any number of reasons why the right lower lobe might collapse or consolidate. Contrast with this the fact that the radiographic changes in the hands in such diverse conditions as acromegaly, hyperparathyroidism, and thalassemia major are so characteristic that one may immediately make those diagnoses. In most cases this can be done without benefit of historical record, physical examination, or laboratory findings. In fact, the radiographic changes in a good many conditions are so specific that the pathologist, limited to a single bone biopsy specimen, consults the radiologist about his impression of the entire lesion before offering a final analysis of the tissue.

Because bone carries with it its own built-in contrast substance — calcium — changes in density and texture, once they occur, are readily visible even to the untrained eye.

You will first encounter, in Part I, a series of pagespreads having problems, usually related, along with some clinical data. Each of these will be followed by answer pagespreads supplying comparable normals.

Part II will introduce you to an additional technique for learning, which we like to call "comparison shopping." This is an extension of the procedure in Part I, but instead of comparing a single normal with a single abnormal film, here we will offer you a number of radiographs of the same region, so that you can observe the tremendous range of roentgen changes that may occur. From this type of comparison you can appreciate rapid changes which even a radiologist might not see during the course of many months of routine daily work.

Part III will be a somewhat more didactic consideration of the fascinating process of bone growth and maintenance. A group of illustrative disease conditions will follow, in which bone growth is greatly altered. Many of the important metabolic conditions affecting bone will be presented in this section.

With all the foregoing under your belt, you will be ready for Part IV, a series of mixed problems arranged in no particular sequence as they might be encountered in the course of your daily practice.

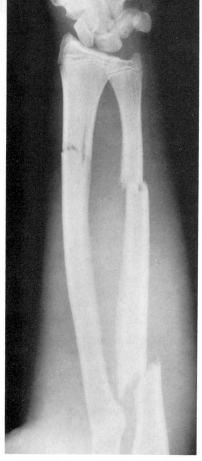

FIGURE 1　JOHN O'GRADY

PART I.
INTRODUCTORY PROBLEMS

These first four patients were a few of thirty victims of a 20-car pile-up occurring on the Harbor Freeway (substitute any other) at rush hour during the worst rain storm of the year. Many are complaining of pain, and after physical examination you have requested the appropriate x-ray examinations.

John O'Grady is still not fully conscious as a result of a head injury, but you note that his left forearm is very swollen and shows ecchymoses. Gentle palpation is very painful.

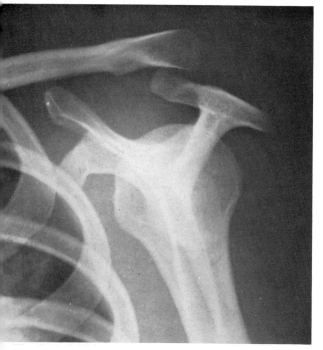

FIGURE 2　HENRY KOWALSKI

Henry Kowalski walks in with his left arm in a sling. He informs you that the pain is in the shoulder. You see a tender, very localized swelling at the lateral end of the clavicle.

Alex Kowalski, his brother, didn't get hurt, but thinks that while he is there, you might take a look at his right hand.

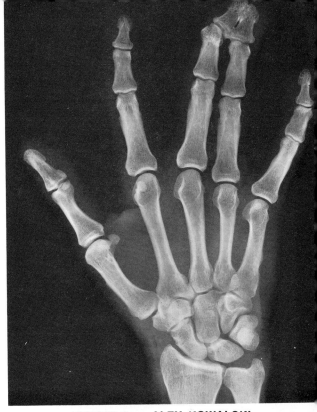

FIGURE 3   ALEX KOWALSKI

Mrs. Joanna Johnstone walks in, limping. She has pain in her knee but is more concerned about her bruised nose. You request x-rays of both the nose and her knee.

LOOK AT ALL FOUR OF THESE PROBLEM CASES AND TRY TO DECIDE WHAT IS WRONG BEFORE TURNING TO THE ANSWER PAGESPREAD.

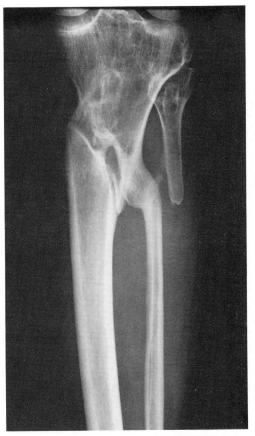

FIGURE 4   MRS. JOHNSTONE

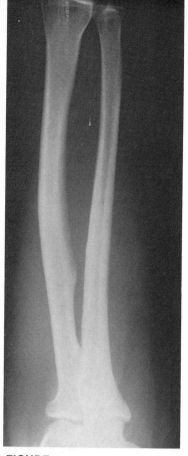

FIGURE 5   Normal forearm.

ANSWERS

The most common and impressive change in bone one can encounter is, without doubt, the fracture. *John O'Grady* has fractures of both bones of the forearm. Fractures, as traumatic interruptions in the continuity of bone, have a wide range of x-ray appearance, some of which you will encounter later in the series of exercises. Is Figure 5 *John O'Grady's* other forearm? (Answer in box on Page 5.)

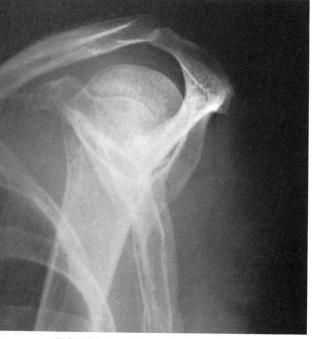

FIGURE 6   Normal shoulder.

Figure 6 is *Henry Kowalski's* uninjured shoulder (photographically reversed) for comparison. Figure 2 shows no fracture—no interruption of bone. But there *is* an abnormality of positional relationship of one bone to another—an acromioclavicular dislocation.

> *TO MAKE DIRECT COMPARISON OF ONE FILM WITH ANOTHER, PLACE THE MARGIN OF PAGE 4 IN THE CENTER OF PAGE 2. YOU MAY USE THIS METHOD THROUGHOUT THE BOOK.*

Alex Kowalski's other hand was normal. It was obvious from your clinical examination that he had a congenital fusion of the soft tissues of his third and fourth digits. The radiograph adds the information that the bones are also fused. (Compare Alex's hand with figure 15 in which the tips of third and fourth fingers were intentionally overlapped.)

Mrs. Johnstone had been hit by a car 10 years ago and has had pain in her knee (in damp weather) ever since. Figure 7 is a normal leg. There had been a large confluent hematoma surrounding the fractures of the tibia and fibula at the time of the original injury. As we shall see in other fractures, the hematoma provides a base for the deposition of bone (callus) for the purpose of healing. The process has resulted here in a smooth fusion of the fibula to the tibia. Note that the original fracture line in the tibia is still visible, though bridged by bone. Can you account for the difference in density between the upper and midportions of the tibial shaft? (Answer on Page 6.)

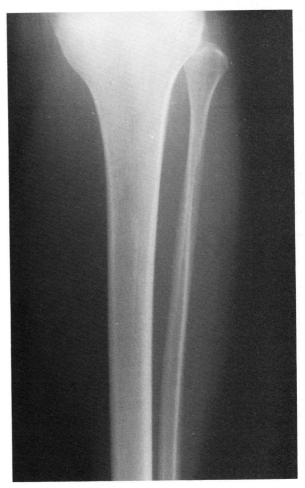

FIGURE 7 Normal leg.

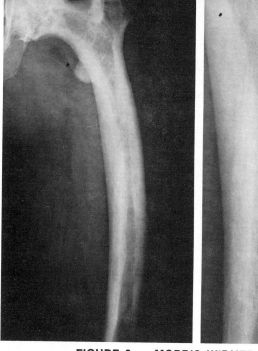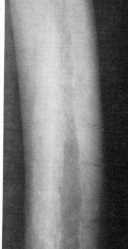

FIGURE 8   MORRIS WIDNER

PROBLEMS

Morris Widner is a 58-year-old mail carrier who has been complaining of pain in his left thigh and hip for many months. He had dismissed it as "a little rheumatism." He is brought into the Emergency Room after falling while being chased by an irate dachshund. When you examine him, you find a bruise over the sacrum and the left hip. Films of the pelvis and femur are obtained. What is the abnormality of form? Is there a fracture? Aside from form, are the details of bony structure altered? How?

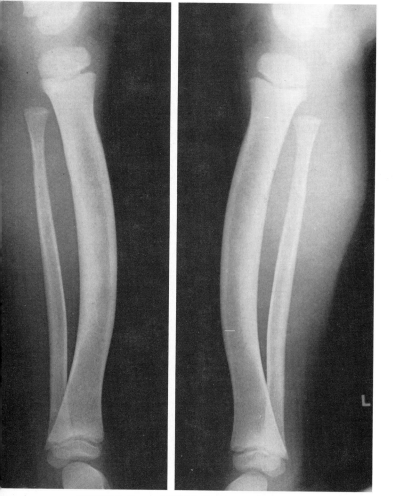

FIGURE 9   JERRY STONER, Age 2

Jerry Stoner has been in a foster home for a year. He is brought in by the social worker because of an upper respiratory infection, but you note abnormality of both lower legs and request films. The lateral views are shown.

Addendum Mrs. Johnstone: Decreased density above the old fracture is the result of bone loss — osteoporosis of disuse.

Joseph Boos has had a deformity of his left leg ever since he can remember. From the appearance of normal knees you have already seen, can you find at least two specific abnormalities? Can you explain the unusual shape of the tibia?

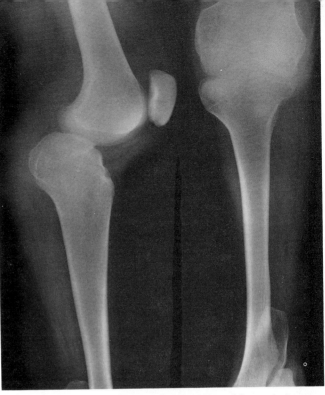

FIGURE 10   JOSEPH BOOS, AP and lateral views.

Jonathan Dreiser, who is 22 years old, injured his wrist after a fall on the outstretched arm a year ago. His wrist has been weak and painful ever since. An operation was advised and performed. This is an examination after surgery. What has been done? Is there anything wrong with the bones about the wrist which might indicate how long ago surgery was done?

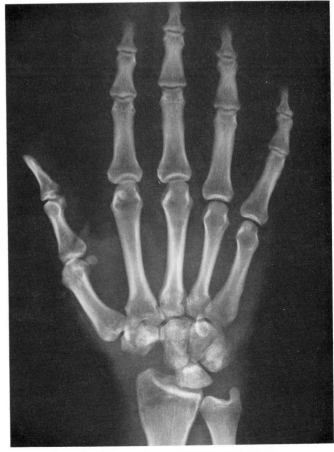

FIGURE 11   JONATHAN DREISER

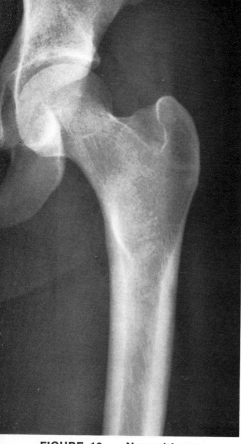

FIGURE 12   Normal femur.

ANSWERS

When compared with the normal femur in Figure 12, *Mr. Widner's* femur is notably bowed. There is also a relative increase in roentgen density of the bone. This is most obvious in the shaft (or diaphysis) where apparent overgrowth of rather featureless compact bone has begun to encroach on the dark shadow of the medullary cavity. Overgrowth is also centrifugal, resulting in a net increase in diameter of the shaft from new subperiosteal bone formation. In the head and neck of the femur the fine trabeculae of the normal (Fig. 12) are in marked contrast to the irregularly arranged, coarse trabeculae of the diseased bone. Because the abnormal bone of Paget's disease (which *Mr. Widner* has) is of poor structural strength, a gradual lateral bowing of the femur has resulted. You will most often recognize Paget's disease in its chronic healing phase when the bone is thickened and the trabecular pattern distorted. Lucent lines partway across the bone, sometimes seen in Paget's disease, are known as "pseudo-fractures."

Jerry Stoner, who is 4 years old, shows symmetrical, anterior bowing of both tibias (healed rickets). Two years ago he was suffering from active rickets. Because of severe dietary vitamin-D deficiency he was unable to absorb enough calcium from his intestine to adequately mineralize his bones, hence the bowing. Note how the thickness of the posterior cortex is being correctively increased, eventually to offset the bowing. This is often called remodeling.

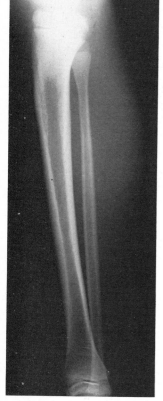

FIGURE 13   Normal leg.

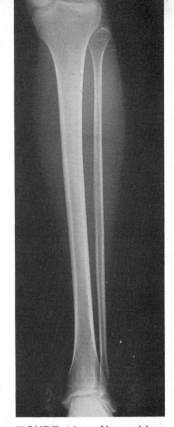

Mr. Boos' fibula is congenitally absent except for the small misshapen remnant of bone at the distal end of the extremity. Though the fibula is a non-weight-bearing bone, it does provide a locus of attachment for many muscle groups. The final adult shape of any bone is the result of many forces, not the least of which is muscular pull. In the absence of the fibula, there has been a marked rearrangement of muscular tension vectors, resulting in an unusually shaped tibia and what appears to be a grossly unstable knee joint.

Acquired absence of bone is much more common. *Mr. Dreiser* had fractured the navicular bone of his wrist. Because of peculiarities in the blood supply to that bone, his fracture failed to heal, resulting in a painful wrist joint. Removal of the dead bone is often the only satisfactory treatment. The film of the wrist (Fig. 11) was made immediately following removal of a heavily autographed plaster cast, which had been in place for six weeks. Comparison with the normal wrist in Figure 15 makes more easily visible the marked "demineralization" of the distal radius, ulna, and remaining carpal bones. This is *bone loss* as a result of absent muscular pull, or, as commonly termed, *atrophy of disuse.* "Demineralization" is a much abused term in common use and it should be avoided. It is misleading because it implies loss of mineral in still existing bone rather than a net decrease in bone mass—the actual state of affairs. Note the superimposition of greater on lesser multangular, and of pisiform on triquetrum.

FIGURE 14   Normal leg.

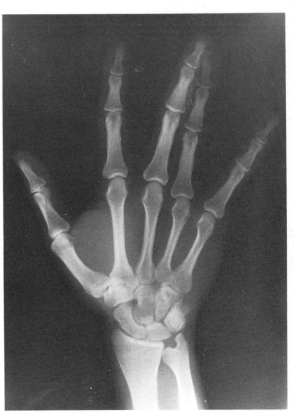

FIGURE 15   Normal hand.

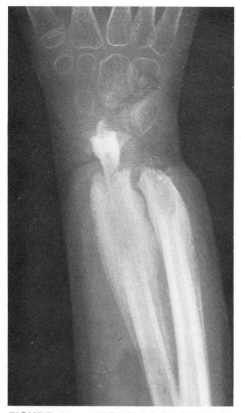

FIGURE 16   NICHOLAS PROWSE, Age 6

FOUR PATIENTS FROM ARTHRITIS CLINIC WITH PAIN

Nicholas Prowse is brought in by his mother because of swelling of his right wrist. He has complained of pain for two months. His appetite has been very poor and he has lost weight. Mrs. Prowse had attributed his complaints to "growing pains" until she took his temperature and found it to be 103° F.

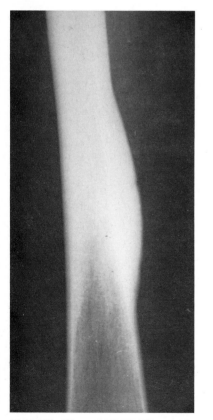

FIGURE 17   BERTRAM KRAMER

Bertram Kramer, 18 years old, is sent to Arthritis Clinic from school because of pain in his knee and thigh. The school nurse feels that the problem is psychogenic because the pain responds so dramatically to aspirin. When you see Bertram, he complains to you that he has not had a good night's sleep in two months because the pain is so severe at night.

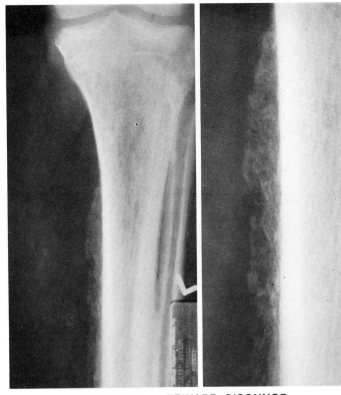

FIGURE 18   EDWARD O'CONNOR

Mr. Edward O'Connor is a traveling salesman. He has been noting increasing deep pain in the forearms and both lower legs for about a month. He says his mother had rheumatoid arthritis, and he wonders if he might be developing the same condition. As part of the medical history, you discover that he is a chain smoker and has a persistent cough.

James Finchley reports to Arthritis Clinic because his shoulder pain (following a basketball injury two months ago) has not subsided.

QUESTION: DO ANY OF THESE PATIENTS HAVE ANY FORM OF ARTHRITIS? IN WHICH PATIENTS IS THERE BONE IN AN UNEXPECTED LOCATION? EXPLAIN.

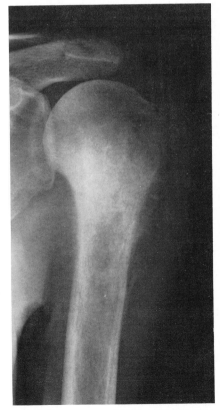

FIGURE 19   JAMES FINCHLEY

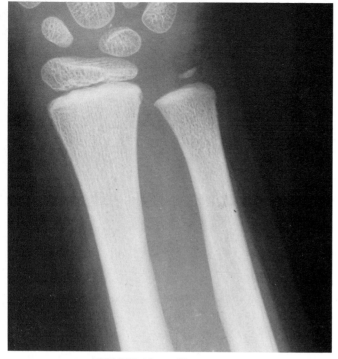

FIGURE 20   Normal arm.

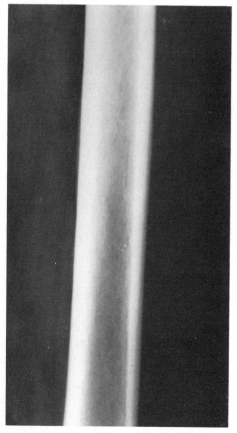

FIGURE 21   Normal femoral shaft.

ANSWERS

As you can see, all that is joint pain is not arthritis! Because of arrangements of sensory nerve supply, pain in an extremity is often referred to a point distant from the site of the disease.

Nicholas Prowse has advanced osteomyelitis due to *Staphylococcus aureus* cultured from a draining sinus which opened spontaneously near the wrist. Note the thick, homogeneous new bone surrounding the distal radius and ulna. With destruction of the cortex by the inflammatory process, purulent material under pressure dissects along the shaft of the bone, elevating periosteum, which, however, continues to lay down new bone. As the processes of periosteal elevation and new bone formation occur at approximately equal rates, a uniform collar (*involucrum*) about the affected bone results. Note also the severe osteoporosis (bone loss) involving the hand and wrist. Note the small dense fragment near the end of the radius. Having been stripped of its blood supply by the destructive inflammatory process, this piece of bone is, therefore, dead and metabolically inactive. It cannot, then, lose its mineral. It retains its original density and is called a *sequestrum*.

It is a well-known fact that an acute infection of bone does not manifest itself radiographically as destruction for as long as two to three weeks.

Bertram Kramer is not a hypochondriac. He has an *osteoid osteoma*. His history of marked salutary response to aspirin and increase in pain at night is quite characteristic. Also typical is the tremendous dense periosteal bone overgrowth. The "tumor" itself is usually a very small radiolucent nidus and often cannot be seen because of the density of the overlying bone.

Mr. O'Connor's bone films, of which Figure 18 is only a sample, excited considerable interest in the Clinic and landed him in the hospital. His admission chest film is shown in Figure 22. Similar bone changes were seen in the forearm films. He also had minimal clubbing of the fingers. Again we have new bone arising from the periosteum, though this time it is filmy and "soft" in character. This is typical of a condition of obscure etiology called "hypertrophic osteoarthropathy." It can be associated with either pulmonary tumors or inflammatory disease of the lung.

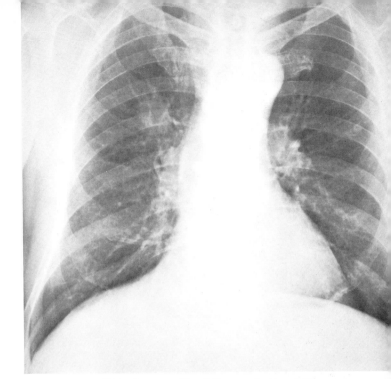

FIGURE 22   **Mr. O'Connor's chest film.**

James Finchley's problem is somewhat different. Though there is evidence of elevation of periosteum at the distal end of the lesion, resulting in periosteal new bone of the type already seen, there are also innumerable, fine, linear spicules of bone arranged perpendicularly to the shaft of the humerus. This is periosteal new bone forming along fibrous bands (Sharpey's fibers) extending between periosteum and cortex. This type of periosteal response is usually caused by a rapidly growing malignant tumor of bone. The increased density within the shaft itself is a result of mineralizing new tumor bone filling in the marrow spaces. This gives the tumor its name of "osteogenic sarcoma."

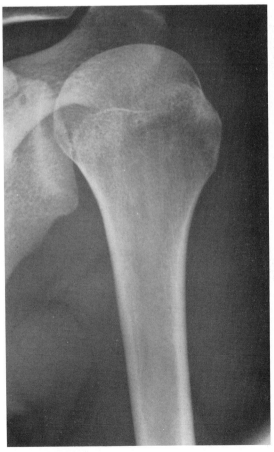

FIGURE 23   **Normal humerus.**

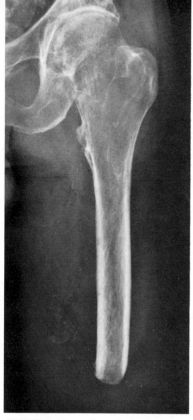

FIGURE 24   L. JOHN SILVER

BONE LOSS PROBLEMS

The strength of bone depends upon two kinds of bony materials: (1) tough, pliable girders of collagen protein, called matrix, upon which (2) a "concrete" of calcium and phosphate is deposited, affording rigidity to the whole. When matrix fails to form, or is lost from previously normal bone, the condition known as *osteoporosis* is present. To carry our architectural analogy a bit further, it would be unthinkable to build a high-rise apartment building out of concrete without first establishing a resilient framework of structural steel. Bones with reduced amounts of matrix are weak and subject to fracture because of the absence of sufficient amounts of both mineral and collagen. In the continuous normal metabolic process of production and destruction of bone, an imbalance favoring destruction may be brought about by a number of clinical conditions. The patients described here are a few examples.

Mr. L. John Silver is a retired seaman who lost his leg during a privateering expedition off the coast of Hispaniola. He has worn an unusual wooden peg leg for years until recently, when the skin covering his stump began to break down. He is now confined to a wheelchair.

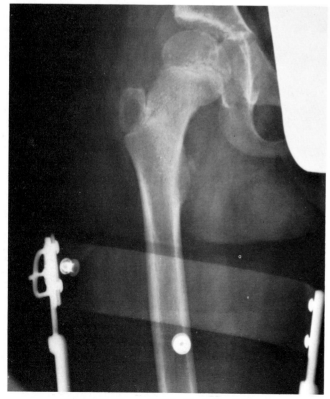

FIGURE 25   MISS McGILLICUDDY

Hilda McGillicuddy has a brace on her right leg. The leg has been weak as the result of poliomyelitis in early childhood.

Mrs. Parmelia Plunkett fractured her femur in an auto accident. Because she is 77 years old, the usual treatment of prolonged immobilization was not likely to be successful. Her physician elected to insert an intramedullary rod. She continues to complain of severe pain and refuses to move her leg.

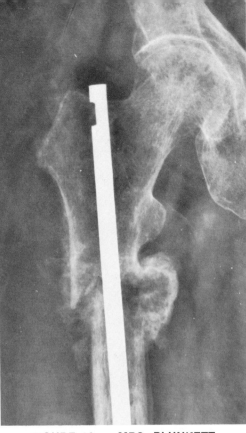

FIGURE 26   MRS. PLUNKETT

Mr. Hong Wah is a restaurateur who has just had his fifth episode of renal colic. After recording the history, you request serum calcium and phosphorus determinations. You discover his calcium to be normal and his phosphorus to be markedly depressed. You then obtain films of his hands and other parts of his skeleton.

(1) CAN YOU DETERMINE A COMMON BASIS FOR THE OSTEOPOROSIS IN THREE OF THE FOUR PATIENTS PRESENTED HERE? (2) WHICH THREE? (3) WHAT HAS HAPPENED TO CORTICAL BONE IN EACH CASE? TO SPONGY BONE? TO THE PERIOSTEUM? (4) CAN YOU FIND ANY OTHER ABNORMALITIES?

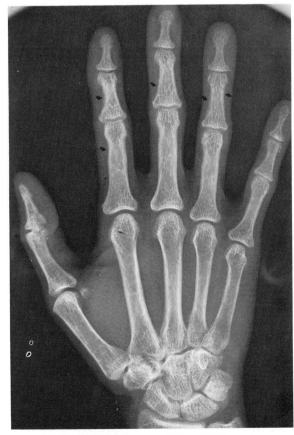

FIGURE 27   MR. HONG

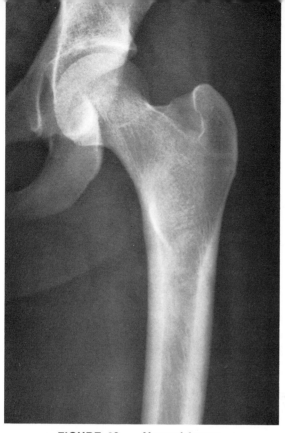

FIGURE 28   Normal femur.

ANSWERS

Although the histories differ, *Mr. Silver's* stump, *Hilda McGillicuddy's* right leg, and *Mrs. Plunkett's* femur are osteoporotic because of disuse. These three patients illustrate the fact that bone put to rest for any reason whatsoever will soon show a net loss of matrix along with its minerals. As is clearly seen in *Mr. Silver's* stump, the loss of bone is not uniform throughout. The cortex of the femoral shaft is thin, and its delimitation from spongiosa is less sharp. There is a patchy, irregular loss of roentgen density in both cortex and spongy bone, where whole chunks of matrix and mineral have been resorbed. On histologic examination, the bone that is left would appear quite normal. The marked shortening and broadening of the femoral neck in Figure 24 is undoubtedly due to an old healed fracture.

Hilda McGillicuddy's polio has markedly reduced the functioning muscle mass in her entire right lower extremity. In the absence of muscle pull, there is not only osteoporosis but also underdevelopment. For example, compare directly the capital femoral epiphysis on the normal left side (Fig. 29). Also note the hypoplasia of the right hemipelvis.

FIGURE 29   Hilda's other leg.

Mrs. Plunkett's fracture shows exuberant callus formation. Again, the typical changes of osteoporosis are present in the bone on either side of the fracture itself. Note, in addition, the unusual combination of filmy (laterally) and smooth (medially) periosteal reaction—undoubtedly related to the hemorrhage following trauma. (There are many artifacts overlying the soft tissues.)

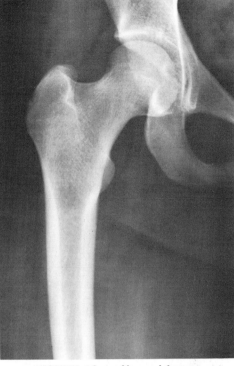

FIGURE 30   Normal femur.

Mr. Hong's problem is entirely different. He has not been injured; he has no loss of neuromuscular power; he leads an active life; yet he is losing bone. Though we have warned you against accepting any fixed combination of roentgen findings as being typical of any particular disease, here you may throw caution to the winds and exclaim, "Hyperparathyroidism!"—for these roentgen findings are truly pathognomonic. In addition to cortical thinning, coarsening, and reduction in the number of trabeculae in the spongiosa, there is also a peculiar resorption of the superficial layers of cortex in the phalanges. (Fig. 31, arrows)

The pattern of resorption results in a fine irregularity of the bony outline often described as "lacy." (Figure 31 gives you a detail from Figure 27, with a normal for direct comparison.)

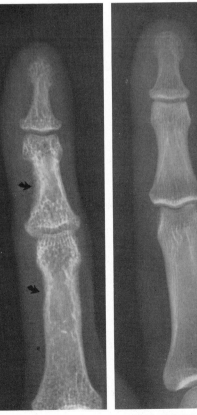

**FIGURE 31   A. MR. HONG
B. Normal**

FOUR PATIENTS WITH SOLITARY LESIONS

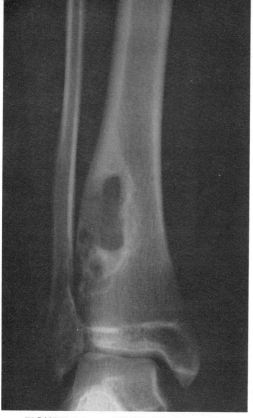

FIGURE 32   JENNIFER POTTER

Jennifer Potter is a 17-year-old who fell down the school steps and sprained her ankle. She had no complaints prior to the injury.

Benign

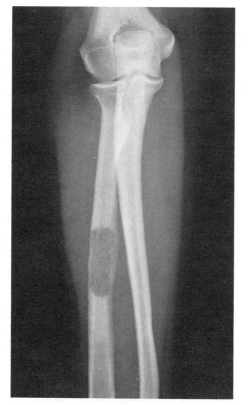

FIGURE 33   RIA GIOVANETTI

Ria Giovanetti, 57, is complaining of pain in her forearm which she cannot relate to any injury. She tells you that her left kidney had been removed 12 years ago because of a "tumor."

Malig.

Henry Darnley is a 35-year-old plumber who has had a gradually increasing dull aching pain in his left knee which he attributes to long kneeling under kitchen sinks. He is limping slightly as he walks into your office.

Benign giant cell tumor.

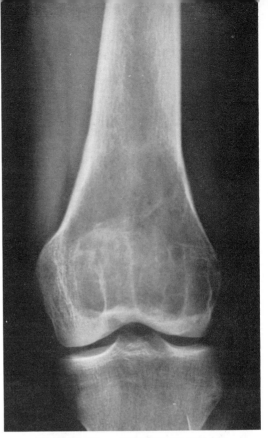

FIGURE 34   HENRY DARNLEY

Robert Dudley, 26, a heroin addict, has also had increasing pain in his left knee. He has ignored it even though it has become so severe that his mobility is limited. He appears in the accident room after having been struck by a slowly moving car. You note tenderness over the patella and a large, hard, slightly tender mass well above the knee proper.

Osteogenic Sarcoma

ALL OF THESE PATIENTS SUFFER FROM TUMORS OF BONE. CAN YOU TELL (1) WHICH ARE BENIGN AND WHICH MALIGNANT? (2) IN WHICH THERE HAS BEEN EXPANSION OF CORTEX? (3) IN WHICH THERE HAS BEEN PERIOSTEAL RESPONSE? (4) IN WHICH THERE IS INVASION INTO SURROUNDING SOFT TISSUES? WHAT IS WRONG WITH THE PROXIMAL TIBIA IN FIGURE 35?

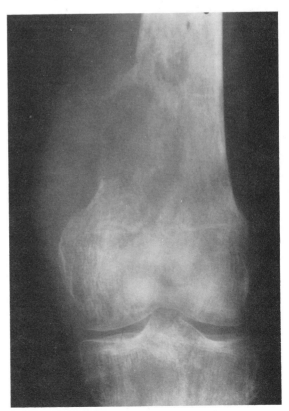

FIGURE 35   BOB DUDLEY

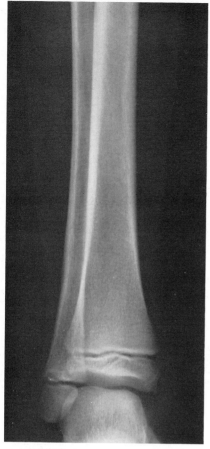

FIGURE 36   Normal ankle.

No normal needed

ANSWERS

Benign and malignant solitary lesions of bone may be differentiated from each other by half a dozen or so roentgen changes which you have already appreciated but not analyzed as yet. You have already identified the lesions in Figures 32 and 34 as benign and the other two as malignant. You have been able to feel intuitively which is which.

Jennifer Potter has a benign condition known as a non-ossifying fibroma. We can interpret it as benign from its appearance because (1) the lateral cortical margin is unbroken; (2) the reparative subperiosteal new bone is dense and relatively homogeneous; (3) at its interior circumference there is a dense wall of reactive bone deposition, also indicating a successful attempt at confining it.

In contrast, the metastatic carcinoma of the kidney in *Mrs. Giovanetti's* radius is growing there entirely at the expense of bone. There is no sign of either a periosteal or endosteal reparative response, which helps to identify the malignant nature of the lesion. *Metastatic* tumors rarely extend beyond the confines of the involved bone. (Metastases from carcinoma of the kidney to any organ have the interesting characteristic of manifesting themselves even many years after removal of the primary.)

Mr. Darnley's problem is a little more difficult. The tumor is clearly expanding at the expense of bone. There is only minimal evidence of reactive response at the distal margin abutting the subchondral cortex of the femur. Proximally, a zone of demarcation of tumor from spongiosa of the metaphysis is present but indistinct. The cortex of the lateral femoral condyle is markedly thinned but not expanded. We can then say that this tumor is more aggressive (rapidly growing) than *Jennifer's*, but radiologically it retains some benign characteristics. At surgery it proved to be, as suspected from the radiograph, a benign giant-cell tumor.

The lateral view of *Mr. Dudley's* knee is shown in Figure 38. There are several notable findings which identify this as an extremely aggressive and invasive malignant tumor of bone— osteogenic sarcoma. (1) The tumor has completely destroyed the cortex medially and is extending into the soft tissue. (2) There is no reparative response within the bone itself. (3) Elevation of the periosteum with new bone formation is seen in the lateral projection along the anterior femoral cortex (arrow). This indicates that tumor growth is so rapid that new bone is being destroyed almost as fast as formed (which explains the "Codman's triangle"). (4) There is mineralizing tumor-bone without recognizable trabecular pattern filling in the marrow spaces of the spongiosa of the distal femur. (Note the fracture of the patella and severe osteoporosis of the proximal tibia.)

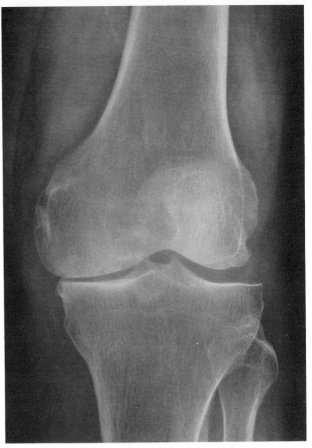

FIGURE 37   Normal femur.

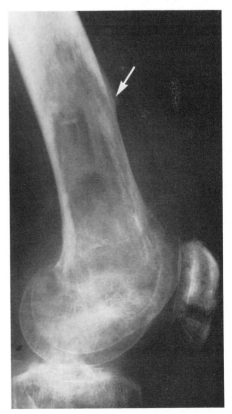

FIGURE 38   Lateral view, Bob Dudley.

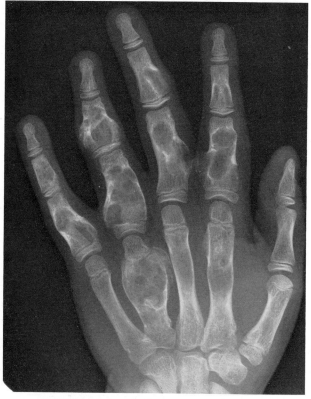

FIGURE 39   PERCIVAL FAUNTLEROY

FOUR PATIENTS WITH MULTIPLE LESIONS

Percival Fauntleroy is 14 years old. His mother has noted some deformity of the left hand with irregularity in length of the fingers. She is principally concerned that a pair of gloves no longer fits both of his hands. His left leg is short and he wears a lift on the heel of the shoe.

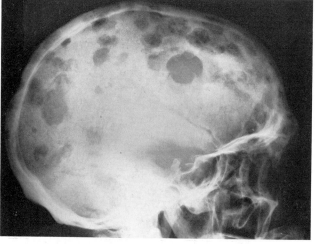

FIGURE 40   MRS. DRINKWATER

Mrs. Amanda Drinkwater, 59, presents at your office complaining of vague back pain and weakness. Physical examination is negative, but your routine laboratory survey shows a slight anemia and 4+ proteinuria. You refer her to a radiologist for an intravenous pyelogram. He calls you that afternoon to report that he feels it is perhaps unnecessary to carry out the IVP in view of bone changes seen on the scout film. He advises additional skeletal studies. Her skull film is seen here.

Mrs. *Florence Megrdichian* has been lost to follow-up for the five years since you performed a radical mastectomy. She now appears complaining of severe pain in the hips and back. Her serum calcium is 11.2 mg. per 100 ml.

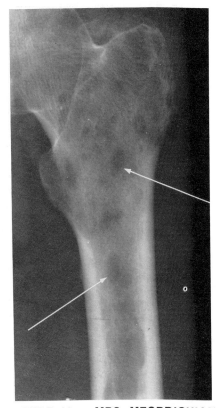

FIGURE 41   MRS. MEGRDICHIAN

John Featherstone is 64 and was admitted to the hospital through the Emergency Division because of acute urinary retention. This film of the abdomen was made shortly after his admission.

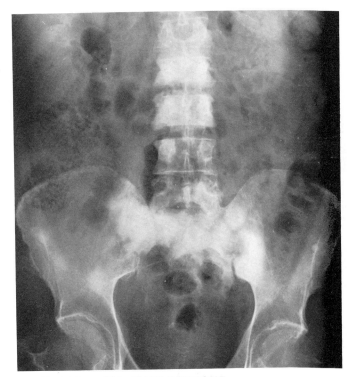

WHICH OF THESE PATIENTS HAS A BENIGN DISEASE? WHAT COMMONLY REQUESTED X-RAY EXAMINATION WOULD BE HELPFUL IN REACHING A DIAGNOSIS IN ALL FOUR PATIENTS? WHAT ADDITIONAL LABORATORY STUDIES WOULD BE USEFUL IN THE LAST THREE PATIENTS?

FIGURE 42   MR. FEATHERSTONE

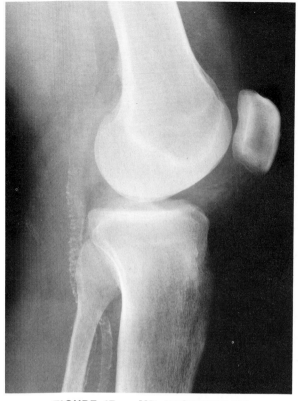

FIGURE 47   MR. WICKERSHAM

THE SOFT TISSUES

Up to this point, you have been concerned with roentgen changes seen in the bones themselves. We all have a tendency to overlook the enveloping mass of skin, muscle, and fat surrounding the bones. You can make up for it only by consciously forcing yourself to view the soft tissues on bone films as part of a regular routine, just as you viewed the soft tissues and bones on a chest film. The following problems are a few examples of the results of this highly rewarding habit.

Mr. Altheus Wickersham has been fond of his morning constitutional walk of two miles for the last 60 years. He comes to you now complaining of pain in his knee but also intermittent pain in the calf, which is brought on by walking and then disappears after a short rest.

Tiny Littlejohn is a steeplechase jockey who was thrown from his horse into a hedge barrier. A sharp broken branch impaled his right leg posteriorly at the level of the knee. The wound was closed surgically three days ago. His postoperative course has been uneventful until today, when on examination you feel a large pulsatile mass above the popliteal fossa.

(*Answer to question on Page 25: Figure 46 shows multiple pelvic fractures: there is dehiscence of the symphysis pubis, and there are fractures of the superior and inferior rami of both pubic bones, as well as separation of the right sacroiliac joint. Patients with pelvic fractures very often have soft-tissue injuries involving the lower genitourinary tract.*)

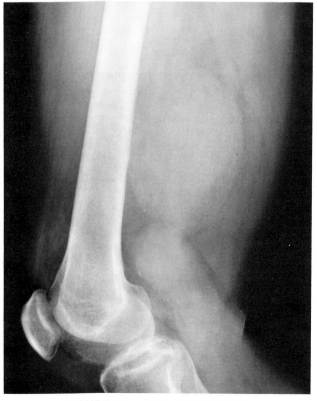

FIGURE 48   MR. LITTLEJOHN

Homer Winslow is a billboard painter who fell from a scaffold, sustaining many injuries. The fracture of the humerus was compound and the wound dirty. He has been doing well in traction until today and is complaining of severe pain in the arm. It appears dusky and edematous, and the hand is cold and pulseless.

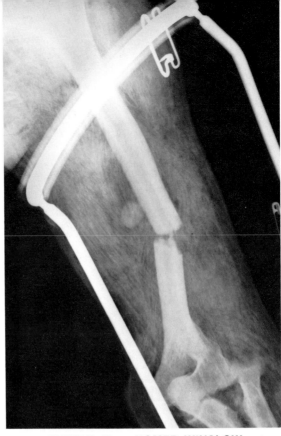

FIGURE 49   HOMER WINSLOW

Dr. Horace Pilchard is 65 and a retired country physician. He is famous for his eccentricities, one of which is making house calls on horseback, an activity going back for over 30 years. He now comes to you with vague pain in his lower back.

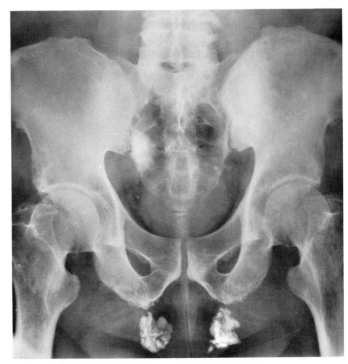

FIGURE 50   DR. PILCHARD

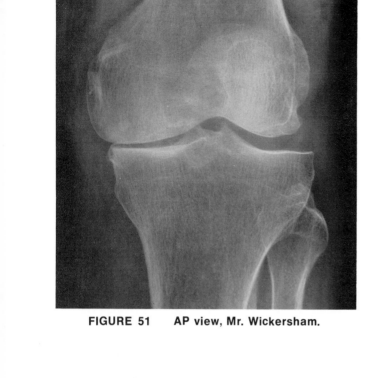

FIGURE 51   **AP view, Mr. Wickersham.**

The anterior-posterior projection of *Mr. Wickersham's* knee is shown in Figure 51. The reason for his knee pain is now clear. Note the marked thinning of articular cartilage and the early lipping at the medial edge of the tibial plateau. There is also increased density of the bone immediately beneath what remains of the tibial articular cartilage. These are the major roentgen features of degenerative joint disease. His calf pain was intermittent claudication due to complete occlusion of the calcified, atherosclerotic popliteal artery discovered at arteriography. (Difference between density of the two films is due to exposure.)

Tiny Littlejohn has a huge traumatic aneurysm. The mass of the aneurysm is clearly visible outlined by the displaced popliteal fat. The diagnosis was confirmed arteriographically, and the aneurysm was removed at surgery. His other knee is seen in Figure 52. Is it normal? (Answer upside down on this page.)

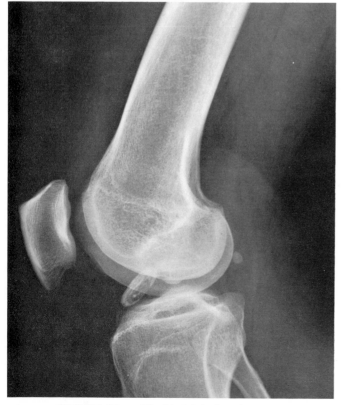

FIGURE 52   **Mr. Littlejohn's other knee.**

The ovoid density seen between the tibial plateau and the femur anteriorly is a "loose body," sometimes called a "joint mouse," which is occasionally responsible for "locking" of the knee. Tiny lost his mouse — almost a rat — (an additional surgical procedure) at the insistence of his surgeon, who had a personal interest in his next race. The smaller bony structure seen posteriorly is a sesamoid bone in the lateral head of the gastrocnemius muscle and known as a "fabella."

Homer Winslow lived five days and was thought to be recovering but died suddenly while being given a bed bath.

The appearance of gas within the soft tissues of an injured extremity and dissecting along muscle planes is the most ominous indication of clostridial infection – or gas gangrene. One would think that there would be palpable crepitation, but because of the extreme edema of the involved tissues this does not occur. Therefore, the roentgen examination is of great value.

Dr. Pilchard's problem is a good end to this section of the book. The unusual dense symmetrical calcifications seen in his gluteal soft tissues were a much more commonly observed phenomenon in the horse-and-buggy era, which, because of his eccentricity, *Dr. Pilchard* has carried forward to the present day. These undoubtedly represent bursal calcifications over the ischial tuberosities, the result of years in the saddle, and are known as "saddle tumors."

They are not the cause of *Dr. Pilchard's* back pain, however. Note the multiple osteoblastic deposits from his unsuspected carcinoma of the prostate.

PART II. HOW VOLUME OF EXPERIENCE IN VIEWING HELPS

If the radiologist sees one hundred films in the course of his working day (a very average number), he sees 30,000 in a year. Most of these will be examples of one of about two dozen types of film studies—chest films, plain films of the abdomen, hand films, lateral skull films, lateral lumbar spines, and so forth.

No wonder he soon develops a firm intellectual impression of the normal and all its possible variants! To the novice film viewer who sees perhaps 50 films a week on his own patients this expert sureness on the part of the radiologist often seems to indicate some remarkable gift or visual power.

We believe that the beginner can often "see" abnormalities of bone just as readily as the expert radiologist if he has a *normal* film to place side by side with the problem film. In fact, we believe that the appearance of the normal is best learned by constant juxtaposition with the flagrantly abnormal, even when the nature of the abnormal is not perfectly clear.

It is for this reason that we have attempted to supply the reader with normals throughout this little workbook, and now we would go one step further and show you how rapidly you can learn from the effective programming of films for comparison and study. By "programming" we mean the choice and arrangement of film studies so that they accentuate or dramatize each other by contrasting roentgen changes.

You have been doing this up to now by comparing a single abnormal with a single normal film. In the next four pages you will be able to discover how surveying a number of normal and abnormal films *of the same kind at the same time* can focus your capacity for analyzing and remembering roentgen change.

Begin by analyzing the film on Page 31. Identify the tops of the two iliac wings crossing one vertebral body. Anteriorly, at the interspace just below this, there is slight "lipping"—a type of spur formation seen in almost all older patients and in most vertebral bodies next to an injured and narrowed disc space. The disc at this level in this patient is slightly narrowed, especially posteriorly.

A gas bubble in the gut overlaps the upper anterior corner of one vertebra, and you will not mistake it for a lytic lesion in the bone. (If there was any question, how could you make sure?)

Note the alignment, shape, and general density of these vertebral bodies. Remember that *normally the center of the vertebral body in this view should be denser than the disc and denser than the centimeter of soft tissue just anterior to the spine.*

Now turn the page.

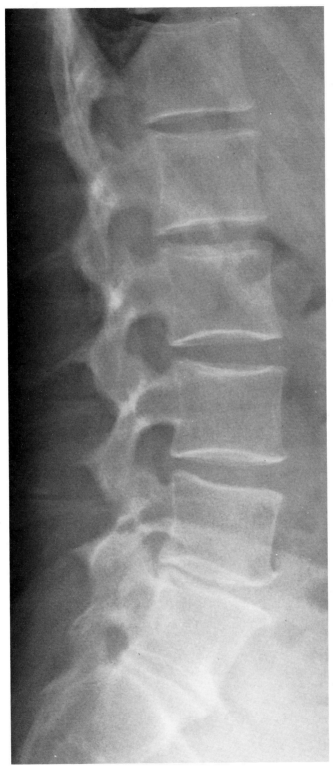

FIGURE 53

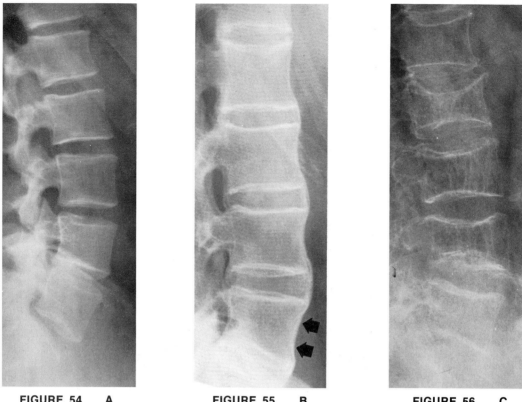

FIGURE 54   A   FIGURE 55   B   FIGURE 56   C

Study these lateral lumbar spines, comparing them first with regard to *alignment*. Has any of them a normal, gentle lumbar curve? Do any show an exaggerated or reversed curve? Are any straighter than normal? Can you see any reason for the straightening?

Now compare them for *general bone density*, not forgetting to determine in each one the relative density of vertebral body, disc, and soft tissues. Now compare the *shape* of one representative vertebra from spine to spine, across the two pages. Then compare the shape of each of those vertebrae to the shape and size of the *disc spaces* on either side of it.

ANSWERS

The first spine, **A**, is normal and has a normal, gentle lumbar curve. Its vertebrae are normal in size, shape, and density and normal in relation to the disc spaces between them.

B has a straightened spine, fused across the discs and doubtless rigid, with calcification of all the investing ligaments. Note how this increases the apparent density of the discs which are still normal in width and shape. This patient, of course, has ankylosing spondylitis. The anterior concavity (arrow) is also typical of this disease, enhancing the resemblance of the vertebrae to bamboo.

C, too, is straighter than normal but greatly decreased in density overall, the centers of the vertebral bodies being almost as radiolucent as the disc spaces and the soft tissues. Note how this loss of trabecular bone mass makes the outline of the compact bone stand out, even though it too is thinned. The disc spaces here are biconvex

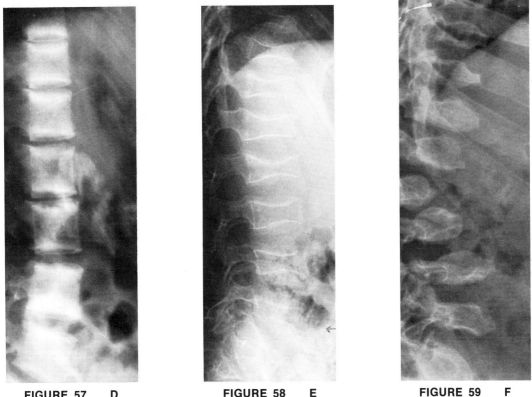

FIGURE 57   **D**   **FIGURE 58**   **E**   **FIGURE 59**   **F**

rather than flat, because the weakened bony plates have allowed the impaction of the rubbery disc into the upper and lower surfaces of the vertebral bodies. Inside the bodies there remain striking vertical bony struts, seen best in the middle vertebrae. This is extreme osteoporosis.

D has a rather straight spine and normally shaped vertebrae and disc spaces. There is a curious dense layer of bone at the top and bottom of each vertebral body, with a lucent area between. This strange appearance has been dubbed the "rugger jersey" spine by the English, and, though still imperfectly understood, it is seen in some patients with longstanding renal failure.

E, a 4-year-old with a history of many fractured bones, has a strikingly abnormal spine. The vertebrae are osteoporotic and flattened to half their

normal height. They are also elongated from front to back and the disc spaces are very wide. *Osteogenesis imperfecta* is probably the least complex form of osteoporosis, in that the inherited fault is failure of bone manufacture and maintenance. This results, even at a very young age, in a strikingly deficient bone mass, with that bone which is present being extremely fragile.

F has a very abnormal spine with generally malformed and osteoporotic vertebral bodies, irregular width of discs, and a gibbus. Generalized malformation of this sort in a young child strongly suggests one of the inherited bone diseases. This was *Morquio's disease*, but the diagnosis is not important for the purpose of this exercise, which is to study vertebrae by comparison.

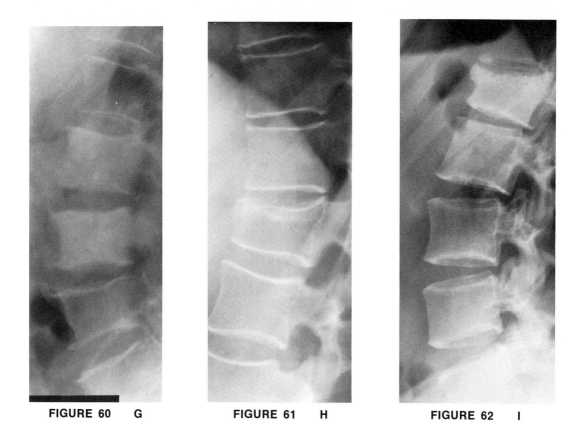

FIGURE 60   G   **FIGURE 61   H**   **FIGURE 62   I**

Here are six more spines for you to study. In these films, decide about *alignment*, *density*, and the *shape* of the vertebrae compared with the disc spaces. Is the abnormality *general* or *local*? Four of these patients had *back pain*. Which?

ANSWERS

(Pain was present in the first four.)

G shows two very dense vertebrae between two normal ones in a man studied because of back pain. He was later found to have prostatic carcinoma. Metastases to bone from the

prostate are osteoblastic and may result in either this uniform density (filling-in of the marrow spaces with tumor bone) or in patchy areas of density scattered about in the bone. Size, shape, and alignment of vertebrae are all normal here.

H and **I** had both fallen on an icy street. In each there is a *compression* (impacted) *fracture* of the upper half of one vertebral body with anterior wedging (decrease in height). The rest of the vertebrae look normal, and there appears to be no osteoporosis (at least of a magnitude that can be appreciated by x-ray). In **H** the wedging results in an abnormal angulation. Note the dif-

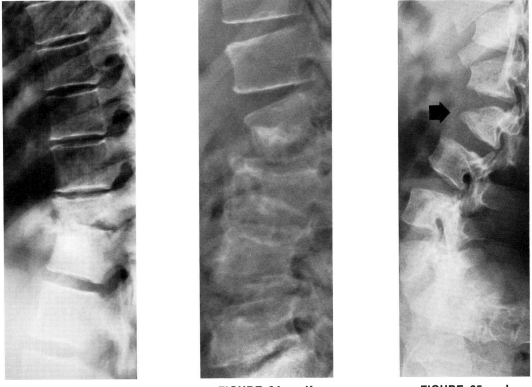

FIGURE 63　J　　　　**FIGURE 64　K**　　　　**FIGURE 65　L**

ference in density of vertebrae above and below the diaphragm. In I, one cannot be sure about alignment, because the exposure has "burned out" the vertebra above the diaphragm.

J shows localized destruction of the lower half of one thoracic vertebra with sclerosis of the body of the one just below it. The disc space is destroyed anteriorly. Swelling of soft tissues and detritus can be seen anterior to the spine. All these are the roentgen findings you would expect in *tuberculous spondylitis* with a developing cold abscess.

K shows two perfectly normal vertebral bodies and disc spaces at the top of the film and then several grossly distorted bodies and spaces below. The change suggests degenerative arthritis, but of an exaggerated sort seen in *neuropathic* joints. The patient had tabes dorsalis. There were similar changes in the knee, also painless.

L is the spine of an *achondroplastic* child. It is hoped that you were not brainwashed by that arrow into thinking the abnormality focal and limited to that vertebral body. All are deformed and the spaces wide. The failure of cartilage proliferation in the achondroplastic affects the spine as well as the long bones.

PART III. BONE GROWTH *(made easy)*

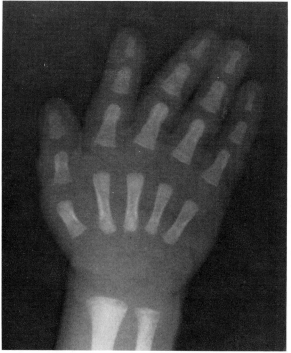

FIGURE 66   Infant, age 2 weeks.

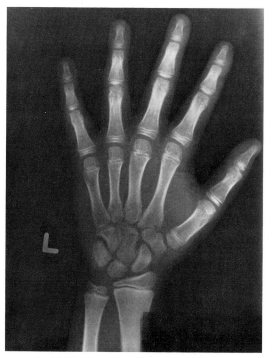

FIGURE 68   Ten-year-old.

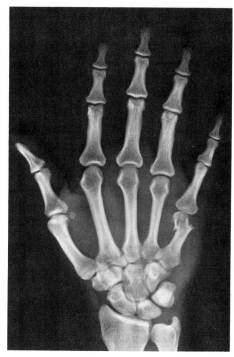

FIGURE 67   Two-year-old child.

FIGURE 69   Adult.

Those of you who have read (and remembered) illustrated accounts of the microscopic anatomy of bone growth will no doubt also recall that it was difficult to visualize the process three-dimensionally. We have no intention of attempting to cover the same ground, but we would like to recall for you certain microscopic high points having a visible effect on the radiograph of a growing bone.

To begin with, study the four radiographs of normal hands on the facing page, noting the ages and the obvious differences in form. Remember that each radiograph represents only one point on the curve of growth. Note the number of carpal bones at each stage. (As a *very rough* rule of thumb, the number of carpal bones you can see is equal to the age of the child in years.) Observe the location of epiphyses of small bones. Are there any sesamoid bones present? Is the adult hand really normal? Can you guess the temperament of this man?

The x-ray appearance of *bone* more than any other organ system reflects changes in growth and development. Of course, chests and abdomens grow, but collapse of a left lower lung lobe in the newborn has about the same *roentgen image* as that in an adult, except that it is smaller overall. The differential diagnosis of the *cause* of atelectasis may be greatly influenced by the age of the patient. But the roentgen shadowgram of the gross pathology is analyzed in an identical manner, whatever the age. This is not true of bone radiology.

A note on the medical implications of the word *"age"* seems fitting. The first (most common) use of the word in medicine refers to the time elapsed since the moment of an individual's birth. You have often remarked about a patient: "He's 45, but he looks 60!", or "She's 80, but she could pass for 50 any day."

You have shown your interest in what has come to be known as "physiological age." Under this there are subdivisions such as "mental age," "cardiovascular age," and, in this heyday of the plastic surgeon, "cosmetic age." During the years from birth to the middle of the second decade, the growth and development of the skeleton has been extensively studied using radiography, and, by referring to atlases and charts, you can now arrive at a parameter known as the "skeletal age." It follows that if your determination of the patient's skeletal age doesn't match his chronological age, something is wrong. Your diagnostic problem is then reduced to deciding which of the many determinants of bone growth is out of line (nutrition, hormones, heredity, muscular development, and so on.)

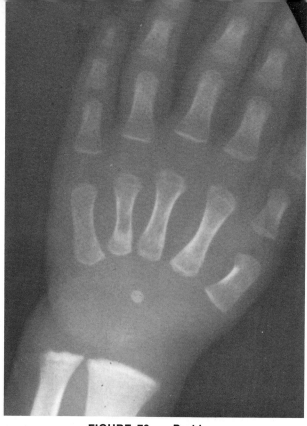

FIGURE 70   Problem.

PROBLEM

Assume that the four hands you have just seen constitute a much abbreviated "atlas" of skeletal development for the hand. Now look at the hand in Figure 70. What is the *skeletal age* "approximately"?

If we had also told you that the patient in Figure 70 is 3 years old, has a thick protruding tongue, and is mentally retarded, you would have known at once that she is a cretin, a child with no functioning thyroid tissue present from birth. Thyroid hormone is known to influence the time of appearance of ossification centers, in this case the carpal bones, and this patient's *skeletal age* is, therefore, only a few months. Because of the intricate interrelationships of the endocrine glands, a specific hormonal lack may lead to bone maturation patterns which are actually the result of multiple endocrine disturbances. For instance, older cretins may show failure in epiphyseal *closure* because the gonadal development has also been retarded by thyroid deficiency. Although there is still some disagreement, most authorities now believe that fusion of the growth plate and cessation of growth result from increase in androgenic secretions (gonadal and adrenal).

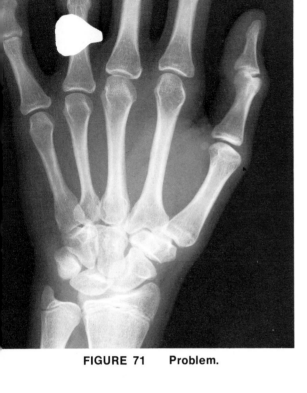

FIGURE 71   Problem.

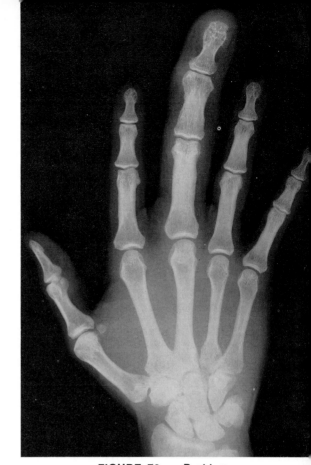

FIGURE 72   Problem.

As another example, the patient in Figure 71 is 30 years old but has hypogonadism because of pituitary hypofunction. The pituitary was destroyed by a craniopharyngioma after full growth (and epiphyseal fusion) of the hand. Note that the distal growth plates of the radius and ulna are still open, however. They should have been closed by the age of 24. (Is the growth problem in Figure 72 hormonal in origin?)

You can see from these examples that determination of skeletal age is an important diagnostic tool. In assessing skeletal age we are interested in several different (but of course related) growth processes: (1) growth in length, (2) growth in diameter, (3) time and order of appearance of the *secondary* centers of ossification, and (4) modeling—the process which gives each bone its distinctive shape and proportions. Each of these parameters of growth has its own endocrine dependence, its unique metabolic and genetic potential for abnormality—all adding up to one of the most intriguing subjects in medicine.

ANSWER TO PROBLEM IN THE TEXT Figure 72

No, the abnormality in the illustration is not an endocrine problem. It couldn't be, since, except for the middle finger, the hand is entirely normal. One of the familiar principles of endocrinology is that the response of a particular tissue, *as end organ*, to a given hormonal stimulus will be uniform throughout the body, providing that there is no local abnormality. Over-growth of a single finger in our problem case was due to a localized vascular abnormality.

Until recently knowledge about how bones grow has been quite limited by the methods of investigation available—anatomic sections and a few notable animal studies. (See historical note on the next page.) Roentgen's discovery was a tremendous stimulus to investigation, because now one could study the appearance of any bone as a continuing progression. Though this method provides only gross anatomic facts, it has given rise to much information of a practical clinical nature. For instance, it is now an accepted clinical tool to obtain serial roentgenograms of a specific part of the anatomy, match them against standard normals, and plot them as points on a curve—an index to the *rate* of skeletal growth and maturation. A theoretical example is shown in Figure 73.

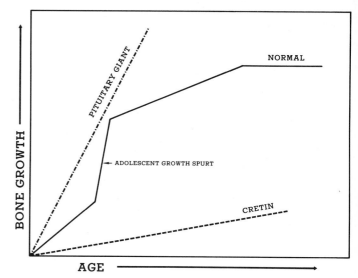

FIGURE 73 Curves of normal and abnormal bone growth.

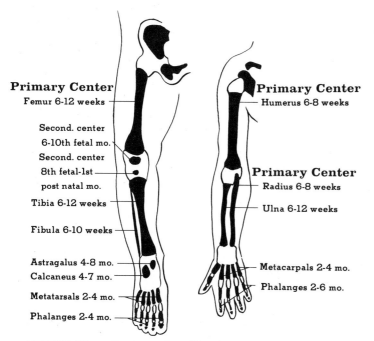

Primary Center
Femur 6-12 weeks

Second. center
6-10th fetal mo.
Second. center
8th fetal-1st
post natal mo.

Tibia 6-12 weeks

Fibula 6-10 weeks

Astragalus 4-8 mo.
Calcaneus 4-7 mo.

Metatarsals 2-4 mo.

Phalanges 2-4 mo.

Primary Center
Humerus 6-8 weeks

Primary Center
Radius 6-8 weeks

Ulna 6-12 weeks

Metacarpals 2-4 mo.

Phalanges 2-6 mo.

FIGURE 74 Centers of ossification normally present at birth and their appearance times during fetal life (after Caffey).

An account of the events in bone maturation starts at the *fetal* age of six weeks, when the initial changes leading to ossification commence in the cartilaginous anlage for the tibia.

These foci are known as *primary centers of ossification.* Figure 74 will give you some idea of the order of appearance of these centers. Usually, just before birth, the first of the *secondary centers of ossification* appear on both sides of the knee—the distal femur and the proximal tibia. Of course, from this point on, growth in length of bones occurs at the *growth plate* (or *physis*)—the junction between primary and secondary centers of ossification.

John Belchier's Dinner Guest

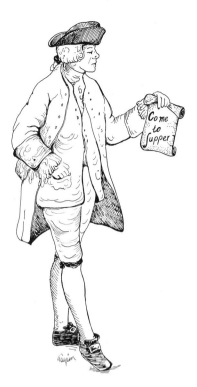

Imagine yourself transported backward in time to 1736. You have been invited to dine (at three in the afternoon) with Mr. John Belchier, an English surgeon. It is the England of George I, who speaks only German; the England of Hogarth and Handel and Dr. Johnson. The microscope has made it possible to see minute organisms, but man still believes in their spontaneous generation! Half of all the children in London die before their fifth year, and the average life expectancy is only 22 years. Most English physicians still reject inoculation for smallpox, 20 years after its introduction from Turkey. Of course, your host is not even a physician: surgeons have not yet been elevated from the society of barbers, and Voltaire has said that of 100 doctors, 98 are charlatans.

Not being able to afford a sedan chair, you go on foot, dressed in a frock coat and knee breeches, buckled shoes, and a three-cornered hat, your hair shoulder length, tied back with a neat bow at the nape of your neck. The company of six men are friends of Mr. Belchier, who has requested that a suckling pig be brought up from his farm in the country and roasted for your delectation.

As he bids you be seated, the servant utters an exclamation at the sideboard where he is carving the pig onto pewter plates. He draws the attention of his master to the fact that the exposed bones are brilliant rose-colored, although the meat is well done and not pink, itself. Belchier demands an explanation. The master of livestock from the farm is brought in. He explains that yesterday he carried the pig up to town and this litter of pigs accidentally got into a bin containing dried madder, used to dye stockings red. He remembers the small pigs snouts stained red when they were discovered. This happened, he says, about a fortnight ago.

Mr. Belchier is sure that in some curious way the stain has "taken" in the bones and not elsewhere, and announces that he will conduct some "experiments" at the farm. It is an era when experiments are performed, even by laymen. You are interested, but not really impressed, being concerned about more mundane matters. You have no idea that you have witnessed an accident which, within twenty years or so, in the hands of Duhamel in France and John Hunter here at home, will have afforded an explanation of just how bones grow.

Up to now men have believed that bone growth is "interstitial" in character, that is, new bone growing within and displacing existing bone. ("Interstitial" growth is typical of soft parenchymatous organs such as the liver.)

Eleven years ago Hales proved that bones grow in *length* at their ends. He drilled holes a measured distance apart in the mid-shaft of a young chicken's leg, and found, several months later, that the holes were exactly the same distance apart. (Two hundred years hence, radiology will make this sort of measurement much easier—something else you do not even dream of as you trudge home.)

Soon John Hunter will repeat the madder-feeding experiments under controlled conditions in a whole litter of pigs which he will kill serially, showing that long bones grow in thickness by adding new bone under the periosteum. It is this recently formed bone—accidentally stained—that you have just been privileged to "see" for the first time in history. Figure 75 shows you the cross sections of femurs from Hunter's litter of *serially sacrificed* pigs. You can deduce the conduct of the experiment and its precise implications if you know that the stippled areas were stained bright red. (Belchier and his dinner party are well-documented fact, not fiction.)

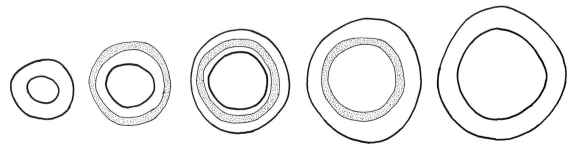

FIGURE 75   **John Hunter's** pigs; cross sections of femur.

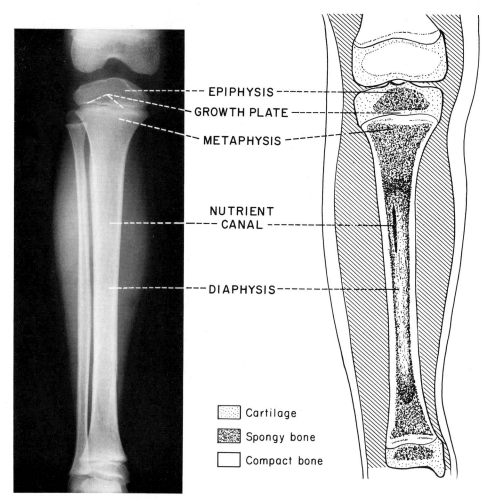

EPIPHYSIS

GROWTH PLATE

METAPHYSIS

NUTRIENT
CANAL

DIAPHYSIS

Cartilage

Spongy bone

Compact bone

FIGURE 76   Parts of a growing bone (after Caffey).

Figure 76 shows a radiograph of a growing tibia. The accompanying line drawing will identify for you the parts to which we will refer during the discussion which follows.

A growing long bone has four anatomic subdivisions of concern in normal and abnormal bone growth. These subdivisions are functionally differentiated from one another. Each con-

tributes in a different way to the form of the adult bone. As a corollary, then, diseases of growing bone are often identifiable because they affect a specific part. For example, in Velasquez' "Las Meninas" (Fig. 77) can you find a figure who has a disease which affects the proliferating cartilage of the growth plate?

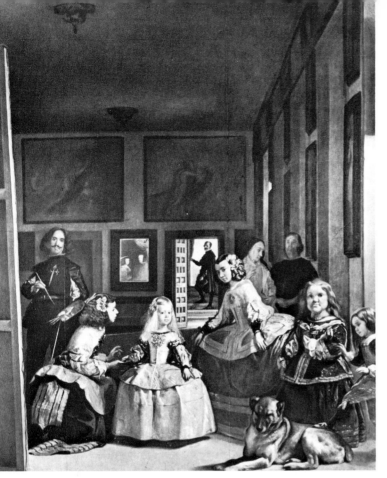

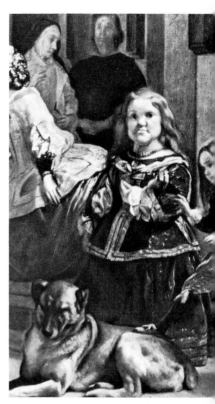

FIGURE 77 **A.** Velasquez' "Las Meninas" (The Ladies-in-Waiting). **B.** Detail (age 29 years).

Much sought after as servant and clown in the 16th-century courts of Europe, the adult achondroplastic dwarf was attractive and amusing because of his grotesque appearance. The proliferating cartilage at the ends of long bones is deficient in amount and abnormal in structure in achondroplasia. The result is a bone much shorter than normal; but, because there is no disturbance of periosteal function, the diameter of the *shaft* is quite normal, the bones thus appearing too thick relative to their length. Figure 78 is the hand of an achondroplast, aged six. Compare with the series of normals at the beginning of this section.

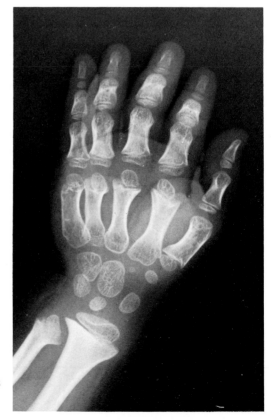

FIGURE 78

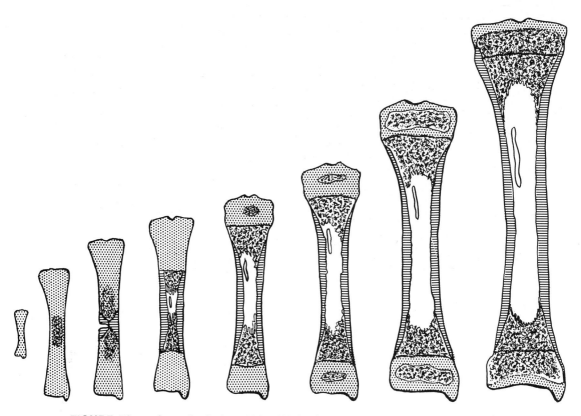

FIGURE 79   Growth of a bone (the tibia) — fetal anlage to maturity (after Caffey).

In all but a few bones of the human skeleton, ossification occurs when new bone matrix is applied, like plaster, against a supporting sponge of calcified cartilage. In the fetus the entire skeleton is cartilaginous until about the fetal age of six weeks. The first true bone formation occurs then, near the mid-shaft of long bones, such as the tibia (Fig. 79). The cartilage cells in the mid-shaft enlarge and proliferate. Blood vessels from the perichondrium invade the central shaft and mineral salts extracted from the blood are deposited in the new bone matrix. (The channel so created becomes the nutrient canal for the mature bone.) At the same time the perichondrium begins to deposit primitive bone around the circumference of the mid-shaft to form a narrow collar. The membrane can now be called the "periosteum."

At either end of the ossification center, cartilage continues to proliferate and new bone is applied to each succeeding layer of cartilage (increasing the length of the bone). As this process continues at the ends of the shaft, the medullary cavity is formed by resorption centrally.

The growth in diameter of the mid-shaft has already been diagrammed for you on page 41, in relation to the early vital staining experiments of Belchier and Hunter. The growth in the length of a bone is the result of a more complex process taking place at the growth plate.

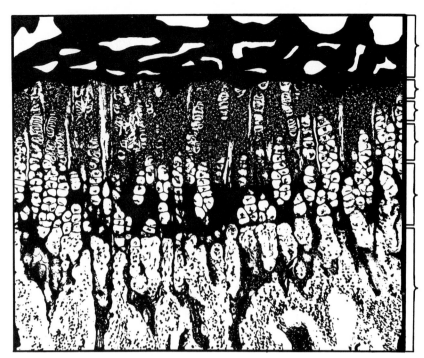

Spongiosa of
epiphyseal center

Resting cartilage

Proliferating cartilage

Columnar cartilage

Zone of provisional
calcification

Spongiosa

FIGURE 80   The growth plate seen microscopically.

Figure 80 is a diagrammatic representation of a microscopic section through a small portion of the growth plate. On the epiphyseal side of the growth plate, there is a layer of very young chondrocytes which are capable of self-replication. This layer of actively proliferating cells leaves in its wake layers of more mature cells, which rearrange themselves in queues separated by amorphous cartilaginous matrix. They then swell, vacuolate, and lyse, leaving an empty sponge of cartilage which has become provisionally calcified by mineral salts carried there by the invading blood vessels. *Remember, this is not bone; it is calcified cartilage.*

This layer of calcified cartilage is visible radiologically and referred to as the "zone of provisional calcification" (Fig. 76). Only with deposition of a protein matrix by osteoblasts on these now-rigid girders of calcified cartilage is bone produced, mineralizing in its turn to form the trabecular struts of the metaphysis. Shaping and restructuring of these primary trabeculae results in a complex sponge of "cancellous bone."

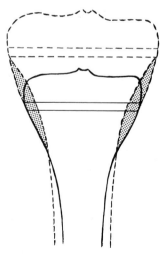

FIGURE 81   The enlarging metaphysis (after Weinmann and Sicher).

The metaphysis, thus, is seen on the radiograph as the flaring segment lying between shaft and the growth plate. It is composed almost entirely of trabecular bone. In the active weight-bearing organism, trabeculae arrange themselves most thickly along lines of maximum stress—a marvelous example of natural economy (Fig. 83).

At the periphery of the metaphysis at its junction with the growth plate, the production of *compact* bone by the active periosteum proceeds at such a pace that the metaphysis is constantly invested in a shell of compact bone. Thus, many of the peripherally placed marrow spaces are also filled-in with compact bone. These processes, periosteal and endosteal together, result in formation of the tubular cortex of the whole bone, endowing it with great resistance to bending (compare the strength of a solid rod with that of a hollow pipe of the same diameter).

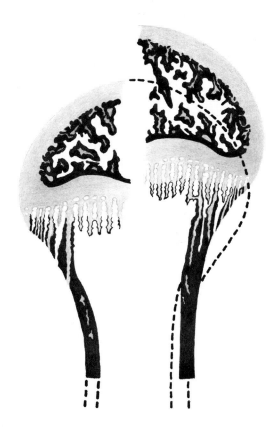

FIGURE 82 Growth of the metaphysis (structures shown in black represent true bone) (after Ham).

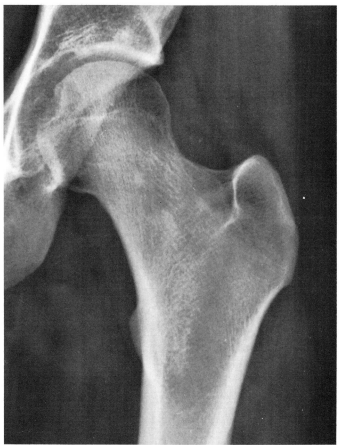

FIGURE 83 Normal arrangement of trabecular struts for weight bearing.

If periosteal compact bone formation proceeded unchecked, eventually a very thick cortex would be produced. However, in response to mechanical muscle pull and weight bearing, constant resorption and remodeling of the cortex takes place. As shown in Figure 84, this process is most conspicuous at the metaphysis, resulting in a gradual, graceful constriction of the broad muscle-bearing metaphysis as it merges with the strong but slender, tubular, weight-bearing diaphysis.

The growth of the epiphysis or *secondary ossification center* of a long bone occurs by a process identical to that of the shaft. Here, instead of an advancing *disc* of cartilage at the growth plate (behind which ossification takes place), we have an expanding *sphere*, the surface of which is the site of cartilage-bone transformation, exactly the same as the transformation occurring at the growth plate.

This process continues until the epiphyseal cancellous bone abuts against the mature metaphysis, at which time there is fusion and obliteration of the growth plate. At this point, further growth in length is no longer possible.

On the joint side of the epiphysis, endochondral production of bone stops short, leaving a shell of cartilage as a smooth, low-friction surface for the joint.

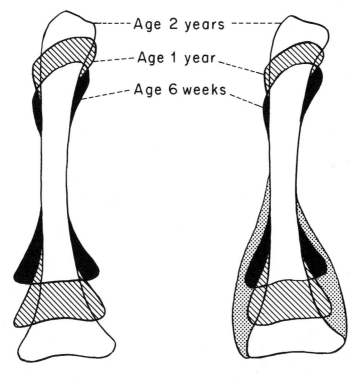

A. Modeled   B. Not modeled

FIGURE 84 Diagrammatic representation of bone growth with and without modeling. The stippled bone in **B** is the bone that would have been removed by periosteal action if normal modeling had taken place (after Caffey).

Bones, then, lengthen, thicken, and model themselves as they grow and mature. No one of these processes can occur without the others, nor can they occur normally without the stimuli afforded by weight bearing, muscular pull, and endocrine secretion. Bone cannot form or be maintained without adequate supplies of calcium, phosphate, protein, and other nutrients.

Bone disease, therefore, is the result of a disturbance anywhere in this complex system. Some problems for you to analyze follow.

MODELING PROBLEM

Figure 85 is a normal distal femur. Use it as a guide for deciding how the modeling process has been altered in both patients (Figs. 86 and 87). (We are not interested in having you attempt an exact diagnosis here!)

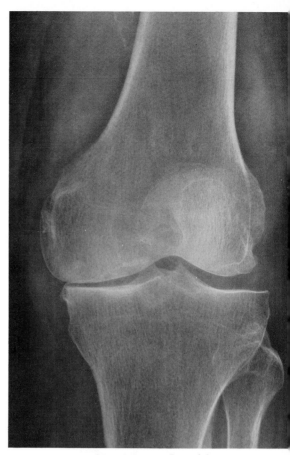

FIGURE 85   **Distal femur.**

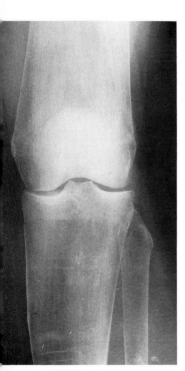

FIGURE 86

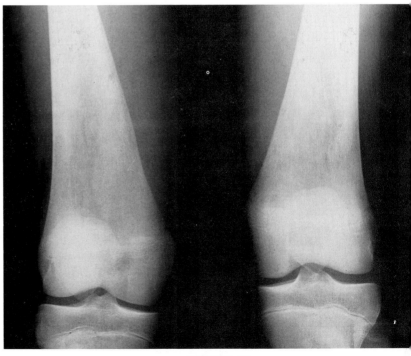

FIGURE 87

ANSWER

The two patients in Figures 86 and 87 had exactly the same modeling defect but as the result of different mechanisms. Figure 86 is an example of an exceedingly rare congenital bone disease in which formation of the normal marrow cavity by removal of most newly-formed spongy bone in the metaphysis fails to occur. The result is the accumulation of normal trabecular bone in increasing amounts, covered by only a thin shell of cortex. The cortex, of course, does not develop to its normal thickness because of the structural strength afforded by the overly abundant spongiosa. Microscopic examination of bone from patients with this condition shows nothing abnormal. The cause is still unknown. (The disease has an eponymic tag—Pyle's disease.)

In contrast to Pyle's disease, in which the abnormality is intrinsic to the skeleton, the bones of our second patient have modeling failure imposed upon them by a generalized metabolic disorder of the reticuloendothelial system (Gaucher's disease). The bone marrow of the metaphysis is an important part of that system. Microscopic sections of involved marrow show accumulation in huge numbers of large histiocytic cells with foamy cytoplasm, containing enormous quantities of a complex lipid material. In the growing individual with this disease, the capacity and stimuli for modeling (constriction of the shaft by periosteal action) are present, but they are overcome by the internal pressure of the ever-expanding mass of abnormal soft-tissue cells. Spongy bone is also destroyed, resulting in weakness of the bone, very often leading to pathologic fracture.

Doubtless it seems to you that these two radiographs are very similar. In actual practice the differentiation of these two conditions would have to be made with the help of the clinical story. The patient with Pyle's disease is well; but the patient with Gaucher's disease has a metabolic fault with involvement of other organs, especially the liver, spleen, and sometimes the central nervous system. In patients with Gaucher's disease you might also find other skeletal manifestations, such as locally destructive expanding lesions, and aseptic necrosis, particularly of the femoral heads.

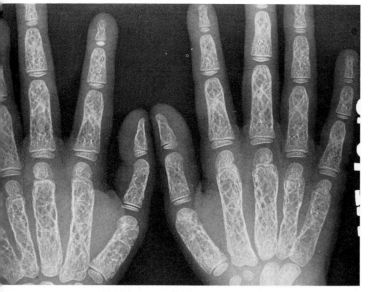

FIGURE 88   ROSA DI NAPOLI

PROBLEMS

The problems and answers on the next four pagespreads should be looked at, keeping in mind what you have already observed about bone growth and maturation. Decide which of the four parts (epiphysis, growth plate, metaphysis, diaphysis) of the growing bone are involved. Then decide whether there has been alteration of length, diameter, secondary center growth, or modeling. Once this is done, you will be well on the way to a diagnosis.

Rosa di Napoli is an 8-year-old girl whose parents are becoming concerned that she has not grown as fast as other girls her age. She is pale, has a large head, and there is unusual prominence of the forehead. You find her hemoglobin 6 mg. per 100 ml. and the peripheral blood smear markedly abnormal. Both parents are of Italian extraction and mildly anemic.

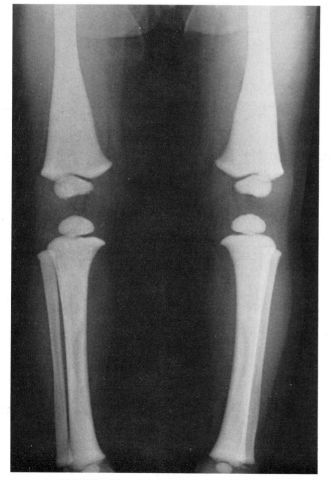

FIGURE 89   JOHN CARRARA, Age 1

John Carrara is brought to you because of a severe nosebleed which required blood transfusion in the accident room. He is thin, very pale, and has an enlarged liver and spleen. Blood tests taken before transfusion show a reduction in numbers of all formed elements, including platelets.

Jimmy Hollis is 10 years old and is well except for being slightly shorter than other boys his age. He injured his left hand playing baseball, and the films shown here were made.

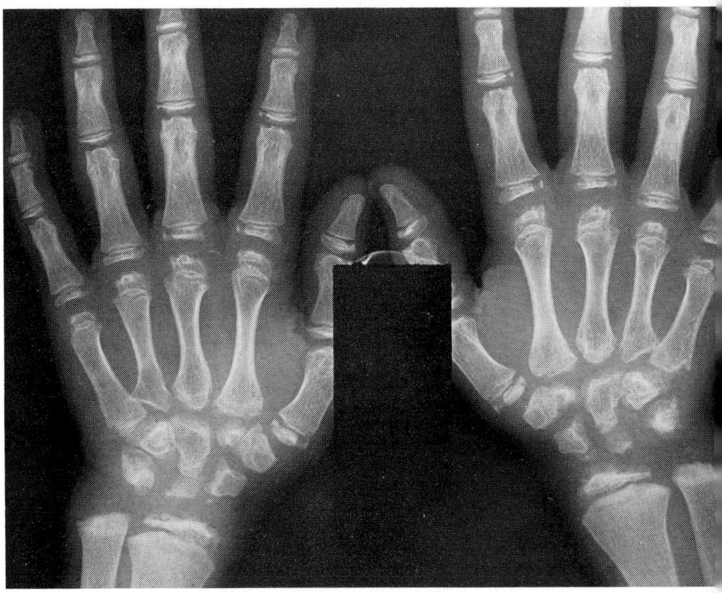

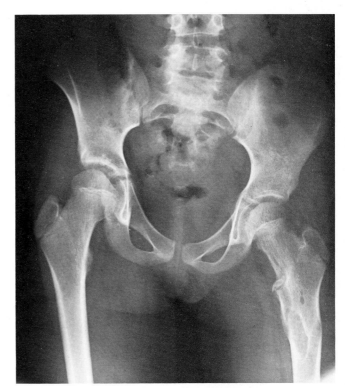

FIGURE 90   JIMMY HOLLIS

Janet Osgood is 17 years old. She is concerned because she has been told by friends that she walks with a limp. She has also noted that her left forearm is a little shorter than her right.

FIGURE 91   JANET OSGOOD

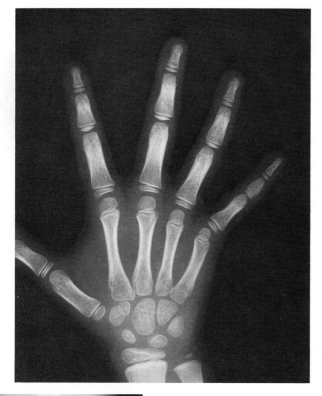

ANSWERS

Rosa's bones appear normal in length. The defect here is failure of modeling—a modeling failure very similar to what you have just seen in Gaucher's disease. The epiphyses seem normally developed. There is the striking additional finding of a markedly abnormal trabecular pattern, with coarsening and thickening of individual trabeculae as well as an overall reduction in their number. All these changes are the result of marrow hyperplasia in this patient with thalassemia major. Both parents were found to have thalassemia, but in a mild heterozygous form. No bone changes were seen in their films.

FIGURE 92   Normal child's hand.

Your first response, on seeing *John Carrara's* films, was to check the exposure factors with the technologist. He points out that the edge of the film is well blackened and that there is adequate penetration of the soft tissues.

After a second look it is apparent that there is no visible medullary cavity in the long bones, nor is there any visible trabeculation. Modeling of the distal femur is also abnormal. This patient has a disease known as osteopetrosis, or "marble bones." It is the result of failure of resorption of provisionally calcified cartilage and bone, so that there is no space for marrow. The bone thus formed is of little structural value and is subject to spontaneous fracture. Production of formed blood elements is removed to the liver, spleen, and other reticuloendothelial organs. The modeling abnormality seen in the femur is also the result of delayed reconstruction of metaphyseal bone.

FIGURE 93   Normal child's leg.

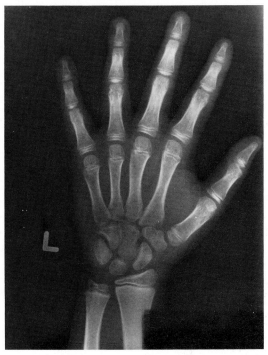

FIGURE 94   **Normal hand.**

The changes in *Jimmy Hollis'* hand were typical of those seen in almost all his *epiphyseal* centers. Development of the shaft and metaphysis appears normal. The disease is known as multiple epiphyseal dysplasia and was found in other members of his family, all of whom were short in stature.

A normal film of the pelvis and proximal femur is not needed because *Janet Osgood's* right side is normal. It is the striking unilaterality of the changes that provides a clue to the diagnosis of enchondromatosis, or Ollier's disease. In this condition, columns of proliferating cartilage originating at the growth plate fail to undergo normal endochondral bone formation and remain to disrupt the modeling and growth in length of the shaft.

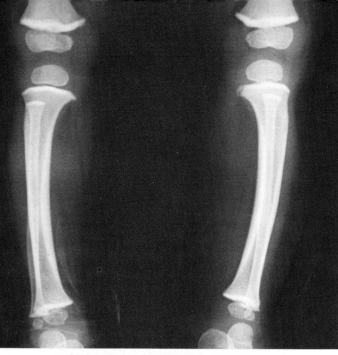

FIGURE 95   PRUNELLA PLUMB

PROBLEMS

Prunella Plumb, age 2, is brought to you by ambulance after a grand mal seizure. You examine her and find, upon funduscopic examination, evidence of increased intracranial pressure. Questioning the mother reveals that the child has the habit of eating bits of painted-over wall paper she pulls from the wall of their very old tenement apartment.

This film of *Billy Johnson's* forearm was made after he fell out of his Jungle gym injuring his arm. You have requested films of other parts of his skeleton after seeing this one.

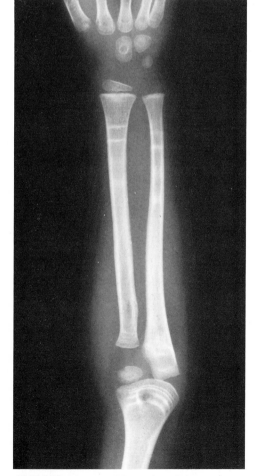

FIGURE 96   BILLY JOHNSON, Age 3

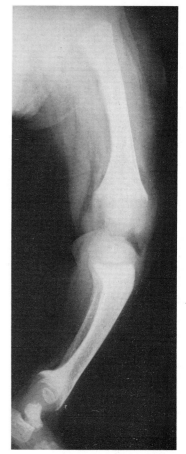

FIGURE 97   RICKY STUMP, Age 1

The two children, *Ricky Stump* and *Mina See,* whose films you see on this page have been brought in to you by a child welfare worker who found both of them abandoned in a slum neighborhood. They appear chronically ill and are severely malnourished. *Ricky* has lower extremities which are laterally bowed. You note tender swelling just beneath the skin of the thorax at the costochondral junctions. *Mina's* skin is covered with large and small ecchymoses. You prove increased capillary fragility by a tourniquet test.

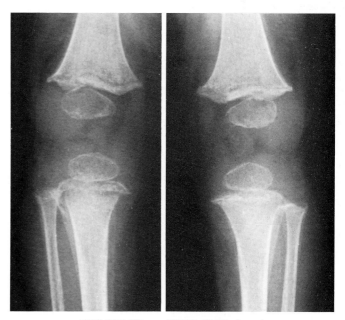

FIGURE 98   MINA SEE, Age 1

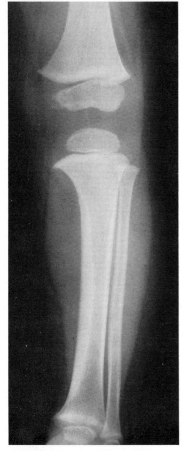

FIGURE 99   Normal leg, two years.

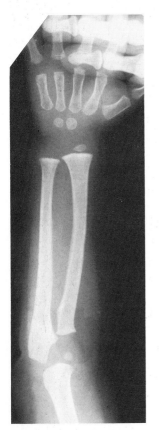

FIGURE 100   Normal forearm.

ANSWERS

Prunella's bones show a very wide, very dense transverse line in the metaphysis, the location of which corresponds to the normally somewhat dense zone of provisional calcification seen in a normal growing bone. (Compare with Figure 99.) Ingested metallic lead interferes with the process of replacement of provisionally calcified bars of cartilage by endosteal bone, resulting in a disc of compact calcified cartilage which grows thicker as long as environmental exposure to lead continues. Although a small amount of lead is deposited in the same region, it is not sufficient to result in a significant increase in roentgen density. *Prunella's* diagnosis was confirmed by a serum lead determination.

After much questioning of *Billy's* parents you discover that he is left with his elderly grandmother for a long weekend occasionally. This good woman, convinced that the child was undernourished, dosed him heavily from a large and ancient bottle of phosphorylated cod liver oil. The dense metaphyseal bands caused by ingestion of phosphorus are indistinguishable from those caused by lead. Pathologically, they are quite different, however. Phosphorus poisoning results in an increased number of true bony trabeculae in the metaphyseal spongiosa. We show you this case because it dramatically illustrates the progression down the shaft of bone formed at any given time. The distance between the dense bands is an indication of the rate of growth: obviously the lower radius is growing much more rapidly than the lower humerus.

In Figure 101, you see *Ricky Stump's* leg many weeks later following treatment with vitamin D. In the active phase of rickets the growth plate continues to proliferate forming masses of cartilage which, because of lack of calcium, fail to mineralize. Widening of the radiolucent growth plate results (compare Figure 97 directly with the same area in Figure 101). The dense zone of provisional calcification fails to visualize on the radiograph. Without the strength afforded by calcification, the poorly formed cartilage and the osteoid matrix laid down upon it by continued activity of osteoblasts is compressed laterally by weight bearing, and flaring of the metaphysis results. Impaction of the epiphysis into the weakened growing area results in the characteristic cupping (seen best in Ricky's ankle). Bone in the shaft continues to undergo normal turnover but is replaced with unmineralized osteoid, resulting in loss of rigidity and subsequent bending.

It is an interesting fact of bone metabolism that osteoclastic destruction of osteoid cannot take place unless that osteoid has been mineralized. Thus, the accumulation of uncalcified osteoid matrix also accounts for the radiolucency and modeling failure seen here (Fig. 101). Note that the bowing of the shaft has been impressively corrected.

In contrast to rickets (which is osteomalacia of growing bone), vitamin C deficiency results in the osteoporotic condition of scurvy, seen in *Mina See.* Vitamin C is essential to the normal production of osteoid (collagen plus ground substance) by osteoblasts. Without it there is a reduced rate of proliferation of the cartilage cells of the growth plate as well. But because there is no disturbance of deposition of calcium salts in cartilage, the zone of provisional calcification thickens and increases in density. This gives rise to

Text continued on page 58.

FIGURE 101   Ricky's leg many weeks later after treatment with Vitamin D.

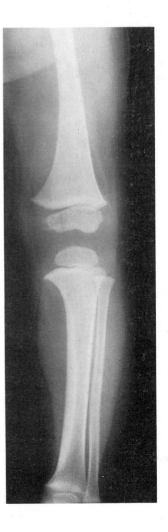

FIGURE 102   Normal leg.

the "white line of scurvy," seen on radiographs at the very end of the metaphysis. The calcified cartilage thus formed is weak and subject to many small infractions, resulting in irregularity of its roentgen image. (Contrast this with the smooth, wider dense line of lead poisoning.)

On the diaphyseal side of this line there is a zone of lucency where previously formed spongy bone of the metaphysis is undergoing resorption, but it is not being revised or replaced. Severe *osteoporosis* is the result. You have probably noted the tibial subperiosteal hemorrhages (beginning to calcify), also a common occurrence in this disease. They are due both to capillary fragility and to the many small fractures of the metaphysis. In scurvy you may even see a gross fracture through the zone of metaphyseal osteoporosis with marked displacement of the epiphysis.

PROCEDURE FOR ANALYSIS OF BONE
ABNORMALITY
CHECK LIST
1. OVERALL SIZE AND SHAPE
2. LOCAL SIZE AND SHAPE
3. THICKNESS OF CORTEX
4. TRABECULAR PATTERN
5. GENERAL DENSITY OF THE WHOLE BONE
6. LOCAL DENSITY CHANGE
7. MARGINATION OF LOCAL LESIONS
8. BREAK IN CONTINUITY
9. PERIOSTEAL CHANGE
10. SOFT TISSUE CHANGE

PART IV. BONE ON YOUR OWN

INTRODUCTION

The material in the first three sections of this workbook has been conscientiously gathered into groups of *related* problems in an attempt to make specific clinical ideas clear. We will now abandon this arrangement for a series of unrelated problems in bone diagnosis, much as you might see them during the course of your rotation in the Emergency Room.

As before, pertinent clinical data will be provided and, just as a good medical history does, will often supply diagnostic clues. It is our avowed tendency (and delight) to make these data provocative — but in doing so we may (as may any of your patients) lead you down the path to an erroneous "snap" diagnosis. You may guard against this by first making a careful inspection in an *organized* way of the entire film, just as you have learned to do with films of the chest and abdomen. We suggest that you make the following systematic observations in each of the cases in the remainder of this book — and those that you encounter in real life.

1. *Overall size and shape:* Are these consistent with the patient's age and sex? If on the film obtained you have a *series* of bones — fingers, ribs, vertebrae — are they uniform as a series?
2. *Local size and shape:* Are there any unusual narrowings or protuberances?
3. *Thickness of cortex:* In a long bone, is it normally thick at mid-shaft, gradually becoming thinner at the flaring metaphysis? In a round bone, is it visible all the way around?
4. *Trabecular pattern:* Are they present in normal numbers? Normally spaced? Well or poorly defined? Thickened? Thinned? Arrangement altered?
5. *General density of the whole bone:* Increased or decreased?
6. *Local density change:* If so, increased or decreased? Solitary or multiple?
7. *Margination of local lesions:* Sharp and well-defined? Is there a surrounding zone of increased density? Or poorly defined and fading gradually into the surrounding bony substance?
8. *Break in continuity:* Particularly of the cortex in profile.
9. *Periosteal change:* If present, is it dense (hard)? Lacy (soft)? Layered? Spiculated?
10. *Soft tissue change:* Localized mass? Calcification? Reduced muscle mass? Foreign body?

Of course, the above list does not cover all possibilities, but if you can reach a reasoned conclusion about each of the ten categories, always using the normal for comparison, you will certainly be able to arrive at a good many diagnoses without help.

PROBLEMS

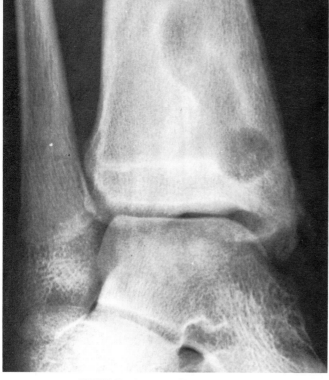

FIGURE 103   KEVIN FARRELL

Kevin Farrell, age 20, is complaining of dull pain in his ankle, present for several weeks. There is no history of injury. After discovering that his temperature is 101° F. and his white blood cell count is 18,750, you order the film seen here. Closer questioning reveals that he had a superficial abscess of his calf treated by incision and drainage over three months ago.

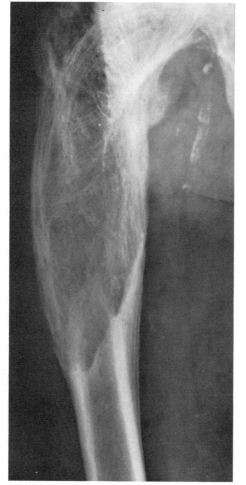

Harvey Feuerstein, retired, has no complaints now that his acute urinary retention has been relieved by catheterization. On physical examination his prostate is smoothly enlarged and firm. Your workup includes an intravenous urogram on which it is noted that there is an abnormality of the femur. A radiograph of that bone is seen here.

FIGURE 104   HARVEY FEUERSTEIN

Jenny Dowben, age 9, has a long history of multiple fractures, particularly of her left lower extremity, occurring usually after minor trauma. She is brought to the Emergency Room, this time because of sudden pain in the left leg just below the knee. Your attention is drawn to her eyes which have sclerae of a definite blue color.

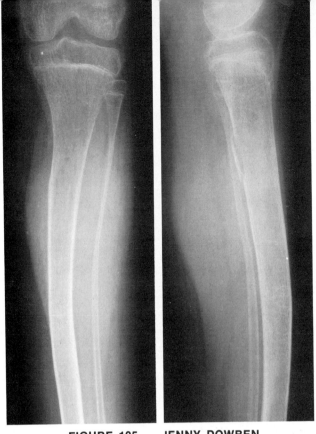

FIGURE 105   JENNY DOWBEN

Raffaello Sanzio is five years old. He is severely anemic and his liver and spleen are enlarged. You learn from his parents that his older sister died six years ago because of a "blood disease."

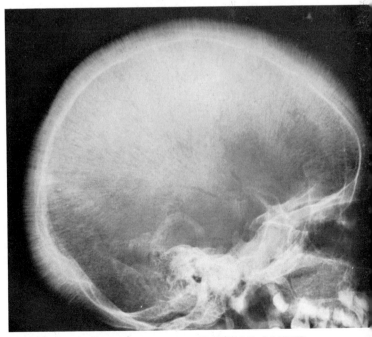

FIGURE 106   RAFFAELLO SANZIO

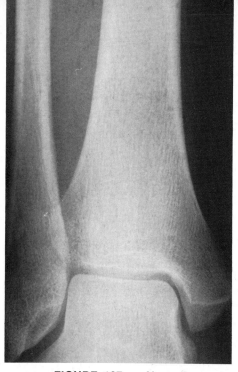

FIGURE 107   Normal.

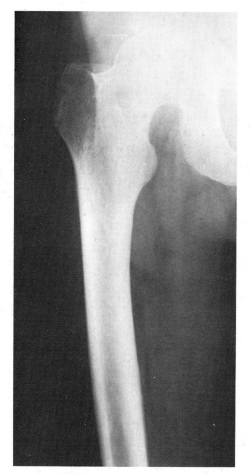

FIGURE 108   Normal.

ANSWERS

Kevin Farrell: When you first look at the bones in this film of the ankle, you see only a curious local decrease in density and some evidence of early cortical destruction along the medial aspect of the tibial metaphysis. Closer examination makes it possible to decide that there is definite loss of cortex in the same region as the periosteal change. You could describe the lucency as well-defined, with a slightly sclerotic border, and serpiginous in shape, which is not at all suggestive of a tumor growing centrifugally.

The historical facts suggest an inflammatory lesion of bone, and the film is an excellent example of typical hematogenous osteomyelitis. Predilection for the metaphysis is classic and is related to the anatomy of the blood supply to the region.

Mr. Feuerstein's benign prostatic hypertrophy has nothing whatever to do with his femur. There is a marked localized increase in size of the bone and abnormality of the cortex that is not a thickening or thinning, but rather a loss of density and uniformity. The trabeculae are reduced in numbers and appear disorganized and individually thickened. The sharply defined and rather angular zone of demarcation from the normal bone of the distal shaft is in contrast to the impression of an expanding process seen proximally. There is laminated periosteal new bone medially, but there is no localized bone destruction anywhere. Disorder of bony structure and general expansion of bone without any localized destruction are the findings which distinguish Paget's disease from tumor.

Bone changes like those you see here are often found to progress to the more typical changes of Paget's disease like those in Figure 8, and now three stages of the disease are recognized: destructive, reparative, and quiescent.

A history such as *Jenny Dow-ben's* can mean only one diagnosis — the disease formerly (and graphically) known as *fragilitas ossium*, now more explicitly termed *osteogenesis imperfecta*. The defect of collagen formation (thus, also of bone matrix) is inherited as a dominant trait. Fortunately it is rare. An occasional affected individual survives intrauterine life, the traumas of birth, and the immediate post-partum period, with appearance of extreme bony fragility later in infancy and childhood.

The bones of Jenny's leg show roentgen changes typical of osteoporosis. In her case the osteoporosis resulting from the bone-producing defect has been accentuated by immobilization for earlier healing fractures. Her most recent symptoms are related to the posterior cortical fracture near the knee. Note the extreme attenuation of the fibular shaft.

(Blue sclerae are also related to deficiency in collagen production. The extremely thin, and thus somewhat translucent, sclerae allow the dark pigment of the choroid to show through.)

The film you obtained on *Raffaello Sanzio* is very abnormal. The calvarium is enlarged and the abnormality involves all the bones equally. The inner cortex (or table) is normal but the outer is difficult to identify. Where the x-ray beam is tangential to it, you have the impression of a brush (or "hair-on-end") appearance. In other areas these are projected differently. The history suggests this child is suffering from a hereditary blood disorder. Your laboratory studies confirm the diagnosis of thalassemia major. The appearance of the skull is due to the marked hyperplasia of bone marrow.

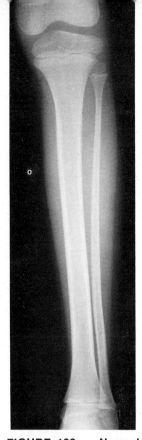

FIGURE 109   Normal.

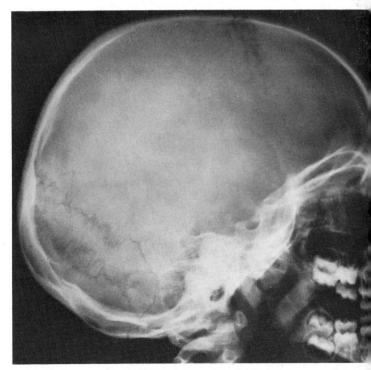

FIGURE 110   Normal.

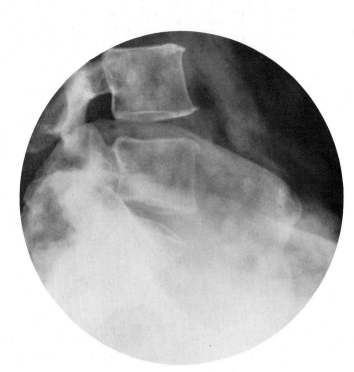

FIGURE 111   MR. CECIL NORTHRUP

PROBLEMS

Mr. Cecil Northrup, 67 years old, is a retired bank president. He is complaining of lower abdominal distention, urinary frequency, and vague back pain. Your physical examination reveals a distended bladder and an enlarged prostate. In the course of his workup, an IVP was done. Changes in the bones seen on that study lead to a skeletal survey of which the film shown is a part.

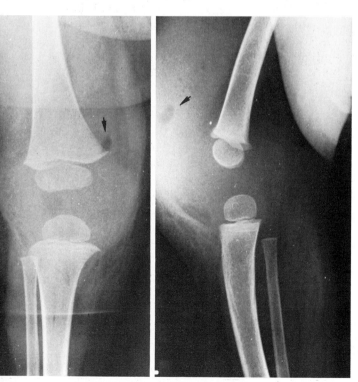

FIGURE 112   CARLOS RIGSBY

Carlos Rigsby, age 1, is brought in by his parents, who state that for the past three days he has screamed in apparent pain whenever his diaper was changed. Yesterday Mrs. Rigsby was able to localize this to his right knee because of the appearance of massive swelling. You note several furuncles on his back and arms which his mother has been treating with "poultices." His temperature is 103° F. and the white blood cell count is 20,285.

Sharon Lippitt is a 14-year-old girl with hysterical tendencies. She is brought (or one might almost say dragged) in by her angry mother, who says that Sharon will not practice for a forthcoming piano recital. After you have gently removed the mother from the examining room, Sharon becomes calmer, but she insists that her shoulder has been bothering her for over six months, particularly when she is playing the piano. X-ray films were made four months ago and showed nothing abnormal. Your examination reveals only some limitation of motion and moderate tenderness over the head of the humerus.

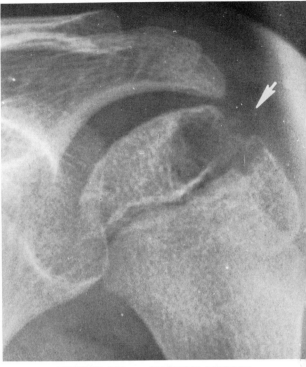

FIGURE 113   SHARON LIPPITT

Henry Sturdevant, 6, is brought in after having fallen out of an apple tree. He is complaining of shoulder pain.

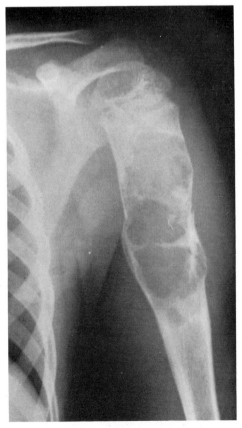

FIGURE 114   HENRY STURDEVANT

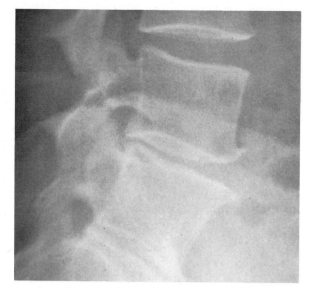

Figure 115   Normal (except
for the disc).

ANSWERS

The multiple discrete areas of increased bone density seen in *Mr. Northrup's* pelvis and lower lumbar spine are metastases from his unsuspected carcinoma of the prostate, proved by prostatic biopsy. This example is considerably more subtle than those you have seen previously. Only a careful inspection for uniformity of bone density will reveal the presence of the lesions.

Seventy per cent of patients with carcinoma of the prostate will show evidence at some time of metastasis to bone. The lumbar spine and pelvis are involved with greater frequency. The mode of spread of prostatic carcinoma was explained in 1940 by Batson, whose name is now forever attached to his discovery. He was able to demonstrate communication between the venous plexus surrounding the prostate and that draining the sacrum, ilii, and lumbar spine. He showed that blood flow was toward the spine in the recumbent position and in the opposite direction in the upright posture.

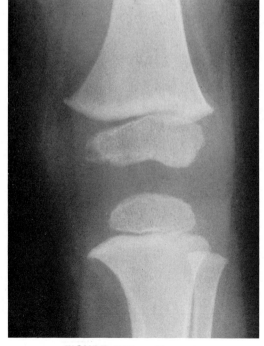

FIGURE 116   Normal.

Carlos Rigsby shows no bony changes in his knee at this time. There is marked distention of the knee joint, however, resulting in separation of the femur from the tibia. The small lucency indicated by the arrow is gas produced by the infecting organism in this example of septic arthritis. Findings such as this in a joint are a true emergency. Prompt specific therapy, including drainage of purulent material from the joint and high doses of antibiotics, will be necessary if the integrity of the joint is to be preserved. Unfortunately many patients with septic arthritis have extensive cartilage destruction by the time they are treated, and the joint becomes ankylosed.

Sharon Lippitt has a purely destructive process of the epiphysis of the humerus. It is also beginning to erode across the growth plate to involve the metaphysis. The most striking finding is absence of any sclerosis or other reparative response by the surrounding bone. The location of the lesion at the edge of the articular cartilage of the humeral head is notable. During the course of her hospital studies a positive tuberculin test is discovered. It had previously been negative, according to school records. This, then, is an example of tuberculous osteomyelitis. Contrast it with the pyogenic osteomyelitis in Figure 103 and review the differences in the findings.

Henry Sturdevant has an unsuspected lytic lesion of the proximal humerus, leading to pathologic fracture. A close look will reveal interruptions in the markedly thinned bony cortex about the midpoint of the lesion. A destructive expanding lesion such as this, occurring at the metaphyseal end of a long bone in a young person, is most likely to be a so-called "unicameral" cyst of bone. The facts of the patient's age and that the lesion stops short of the growth plate help to differentiate it from giant cell tumor, which this example otherwise resembles. Giant cell tumors are usually seen in mature bones.

The ultimate diagnosis of tumorous conditions of bone therefore depends on accumulation of data, not all of which are related to the roentgen appearance of the lesion. Age, sex, sites of predilection, and other specific historical data as well as the x-ray appearance of the lesion all seem to narrow the list of possibilities and ultimately allow a histological diagnosis. The intriguing possibilities for computer diagnosis have already been exploited. Fortunately, a well-educated, flesh-and-blood computer seems to do just about as well!

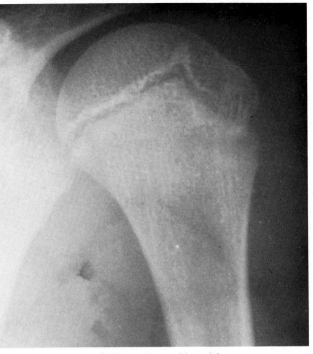

FIGURE 117   Normal.

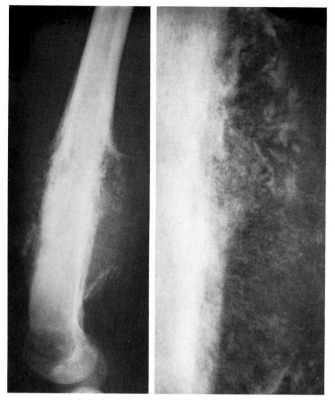

FIGURE 118   THOMAS STANTON
A. Full view.
B. Detail.

PROBLEMS

Thomas Stanton is a 27-year-old machinist whose tolerance for standing at his job has been steadily decreasing because of pain in his right thigh. Up to this time he has ignored a tender swelling just above the knee. He comes for medical help only because he has been threatened with dismissal from his job.

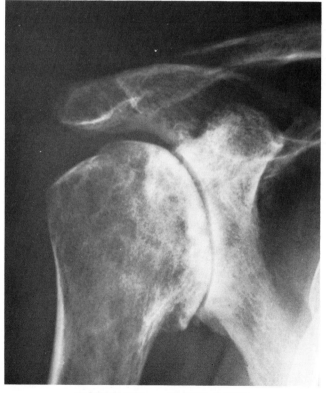

FIGURE 119   ELMER DAVIS

Elmer Davis is a 65-year-old retired seaman who is complaining of pain and stiffness in both shoulders, more severe on the right. Otherwise he is well.

Belle Thistlethwaite is a left-handed painter who has been treating her swollen right wrist with hot compresses for three weeks while trying to complete a portrait.

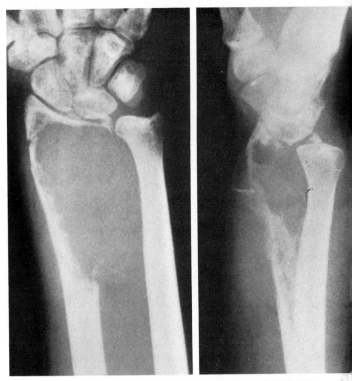

FIGURE 120   BELLE THISTLETHWAITE

Henrietta Hobson, age 25, a black welfare case-worker, appears often at the hospital Emergency Room for treatment of episodes of severe abdominal pain and anemia. Her family history reveals that two other siblings have a similar problem. The film shown here was made because of a complaint of pain in the upper arm.

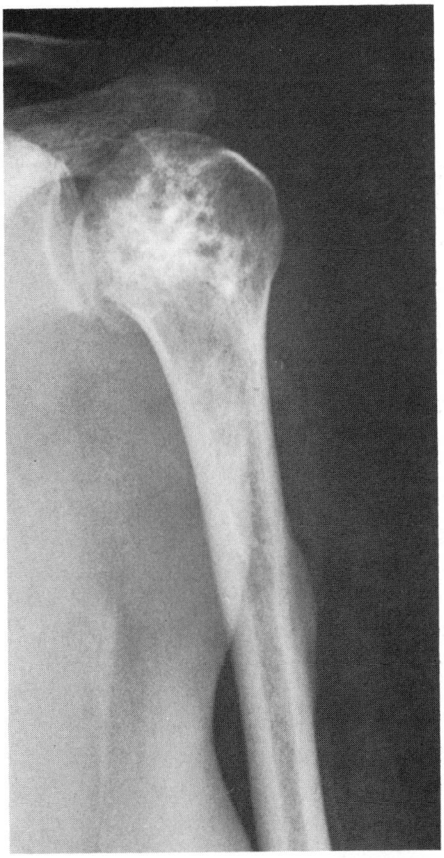

FIGURE 121   HENRIETTA HOBSON

ANSWERS

Thomas Stanton: There is striking localized increase in bone density, along with sunburst periosteal new bone formation, seen best in the magnified detail view. Periosteal lifting, resulting in formation of a so-called Codman's triangle, is seen very well posteriorly. The location of this lesion at the end of a long bone and in a young individual are characteristic features of osteogenic sarcoma. Metastatic nodules of tumors like this (usually in the lungs) show production of tumor bone visible radiographically.

Elmer Davis' shoulder joint shows irregular thinning of cartilage (indicated by narrowing of the joint) and dense sclerosis of the subchondral bone on both sides of the joint. Marked hypertrophic lipping of the humeral head is seen inferiorly. These changes are the typical feature of the most commonly encountered roentgen abnormality in the skeleton, degenerative joint disease. The causes of this condition remain obscure though trauma, either minor and repetitious or a single severe episode, is implicated in many individuals. The appearance of this disease in joints not usually traumatized, such as the interphalangeal joints of the hands, suggests that the disease is the result of interference with cartilage metabolism with aging.

Y
O
U D
O
N
,
T N
E
E
D

Miss Thistlethwaite's wrist film will have struck you at once as showing an aggressively destructive process allowing for no reparative bone reaction. There is clearly a soft-tissue mass present and ragged fragments of bone within it. Because of the abrupt proximal limitation of the process, above which no periosteal lifting is seen at all, and in the absence of systemic symptoms of any kind, this lesion is much more suggestive of tumor than of infection. At biopsy it proved to be a fibrosarcoma.

Henrietta Hobson: The pathogenesis of bone lesions in sickle cell anemia is related both to hyperplasia of the marrow (in response to the shortened life span of circulating erythrocytes) and to bone infarction (caused by intravascular sickling of hypoxic erythrocytes). This most commonly occurs within the small capillaries and arterioles at the ends of long bones. The irregular bony density seen in Miss Hobson's humerus represents the reparative reaction about the lucent infarcted areas. When the same process involves instead the weight-bearing hip joint, infarctions of weakened subchondral bone (aseptic necrosis) often result in marked irregularity of the joint surface and the development of degenerative joint change.

NORMALS ANYMORE

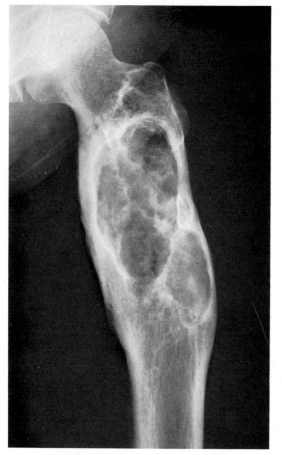

FIGURE 122   MR. GARDNER

FOUR PATIENTS WITH HIP PAIN AFTER TRAUMA

Mr. Gardner, age 45, has had a dull aching pain in the left hip for about two years. Today during a game of touch football he was kicked in the thigh and comes in complaining of a "charleyhorse."

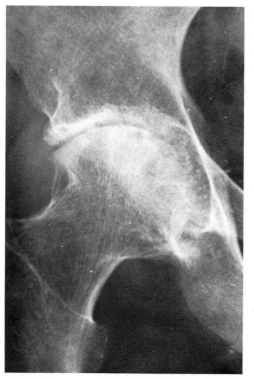

FIGURE 123   MRS. HEATHERINGTON

Mrs. Heatherington, age 50, has been ill for 20 years with severe "rheumatism." Both hips have been painful and limited in range of motion, and her hands have also been stiff and painful. Today she fell in the bathtub and complains of an unusual amount of pain in her right hip.

Mrs. *O'Flaherty* is 68 years old and a retired domestic. She was running to catch a bus; as she stepped off the curb, she fell, with sudden severe pain in her left hip. As she lies on a stretcher, you note external rotation of her left foot and some shortening of the left lower extremity.

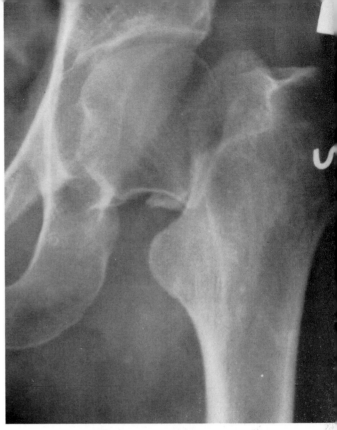

FIGURE 124   MRS. O'FLAHERTY

Jamie Holloway, 4, has been complaining of pain in his left leg for two days. He skinned his knee a week ago and it appears to be infected. He refuses to walk or stand, appears toxic, and has a fever of 103° F. Complete blood count shows a leukocytosis of 24,000.

QUESTIONS

1. In which patient(s) is trauma the sole cause of the hip pain?
2. In which might trauma be partly responsible for the changes seen?
3. In which is there osteoporosis that you can be sure of?
4. In which is the hip joint itself abnormal?
5. If you think any of these patients has a tumor, does it appear to be benign or malignant?

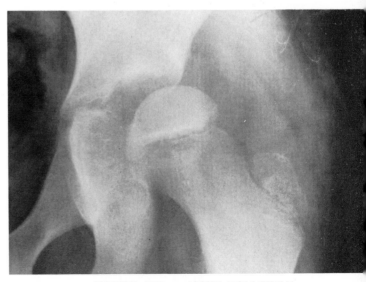

FIGURE 125   JAMIE HOLLOWAY

ANSWERS

The hip transmits to the pelvis and spine the great gravitational forces of the upright posture. Its remarkable ball and socket design affords great stability and a wide range of motion, though not as wide as the shoulder joint. Because of the modified cantilever of the femoral neck, a great deal of weight is borne by the beautiful arrangement of trabecular struts, which is the most notable radiologic feature of the region.

Mr. Gardner does have a benign tumor, an enchondroma, of the proximal femur. The lesion is identifiable as benign from the thickness and density of the slightly expanded surrounding cortex and the very sharp zone of demarcation from normal bone. The irregular calcification within the tumor is typical of that seen in tumors of cartilaginous origin. It is perfectly possible that there may have been minor incomplete infractions (small, incomplete fractures) of the bone thinned by the growing tumor.

Mrs. O'Flaherty has a femoral neck fracture, an exceedingly common injury in older individuals. It is important to realize that, although her film does not suggest it, there is undoubtedly some osteoporosis of aging; remember that about 50 per cent of the bone mass has to be lost before osteoporosis can be detected radiologically. The result is a fracture, even after relatively minor trauma. Tumors metastatic to or primary in the location of the femoral neck very commonly result in pathologic fracture (although there is no evidence of that here).

Mrs. Heatherington shows some changes typical of rheumatoid arthritis (severe juxta-articular osteoporosis, uniform cartilage loss indicated by joint-space narrowing, erosions of subchondral bone). But in the large weight-bearing hip joint these findings are not easily distinguished from similar changes seen in degenerative joint disease (often called osteoarthritis). In fact, without the history, most observers would have made that diagnosis in this patient.

In typical degenerative joint disease, cartilage thinning is the most important finding, but it is less uniform and symmetrical than the cartilage loss in rheumatoid arthritis seen here.

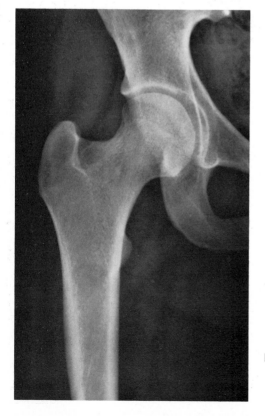

FIGURE 126   Normal hip.

It is more apt to show localized areas of marked joint-space narrowing and others in which cartilage is obviously preserved. Moreover, in degenerative arthritis there is much more proliferation of new bone about the joint margins. Erosions or subchondral cysts may be seen in either. The difficulty in differentiating these two very common conditions is complicated by the fact that degenerative change is often superimposed upon earlier rheumatoid arthritis. A fairly good rule is that if one is in doubt, a film of the hands is likely to help.

There is no obvious fracture in Mrs. H.'s hip film, but minor infractions in the presence of so much bony change would be very difficult to exclude.

The marked widening of the joint space of *Jamie Holloway's* hip is due to the tremendous collection of purulent fluid within the joint, causing subluxation of the femoral head. Follow-up films taken at six weeks and six months are shown in Figures 127 and 128. Osteoporosis of the femoral neck (as compared with the epiphysis) is already apparent. Failure of the epiphysis to become osteoporotic in the film taken at six weeks probably indicates disruption of the vascular supply to this part of the bone. (Compare the density of the right and left femoral epiphyses at six weeks.)

In a film taken six months later the hip shows fragmentation of the epiphysis. Ankylosis is the most likely result of a severe, destructive arthritis such as this and has been known to occur even after fairly prompt recognition and treatment. The extremely rapid destruction of articular cartilage is a result of the exposure to high concentrations of proteolytic enzymes released by the breakdown of polymorphonuclear leukocytes. Therefore, septic arthritis in children must be diagnosed and treated aggressively within 24 hours if the joint is to be preserved.

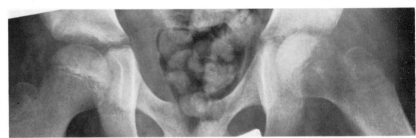

**FIGURE 127   JAMIE—
six weeks later.**

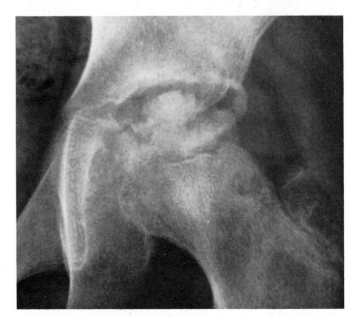

FIGURE 128   JAMIE—six months later.

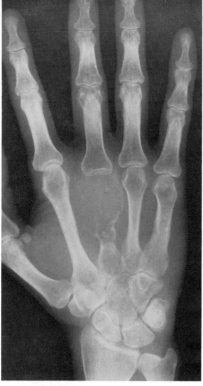

FIGURE 129   MRS. H.

FINAL EXERCISE
(Bones of Contention)

It is not only gypsy fortune-tellers who find hands of great interest in predicting the future. Radiologists and other specialists have often been impressed with the frequency with which radiographs of the hands reflect a generalized disease process. Also, the human hand, because it is the marvelous evolutionary tool that it is, constantly gets itself into machines, under saws and hammers, and into other unhealthy places. Hands radiographed after trauma often show evidence of some other disease condition not yet diagnosed.

The hand films on this and the next four pages should be examined in sequence and your impressions noted on scrap paper. A normal film is included, and once you decide which it is, it will be useful to you as a guide. A series of questions follows on page 81. These are to be answered by entering the appropriate patient's initial in the blank following each question. Correctly filled in, the answers will spell (vertically) what we'll do as you close the book.

Mrs. H is a 35-year-old woman who has noted swelling in the mid-portion of her hand which was painless until a few hours ago. She experienced sudden pain in this area while attempting to open a seldom-used pancake syrup bottle.

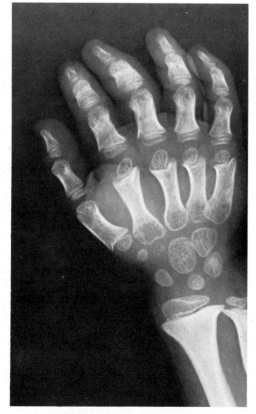

FIGURE 130   MASTER E.

Master E is 6 years old and much shorter than he should be for his age. His parents, who are of average height, are concerned.

This elderly man, *Mr. A*, has been a manual laborer for many years. In the past six or seven years he has had recurrent episodes of severe pain in the fingers, brought on by exposure to cold. He is no longer able to flex his fingers. The skin of his hands is shiny, pale, and indurated.

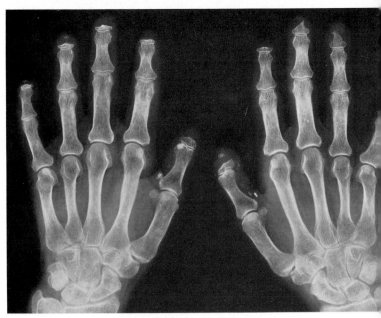

FIGURE 131   MR. A.

Master K is 3 years old and has fractured his tibia without apparent trauma. The hand film is part of a skeletal survey.

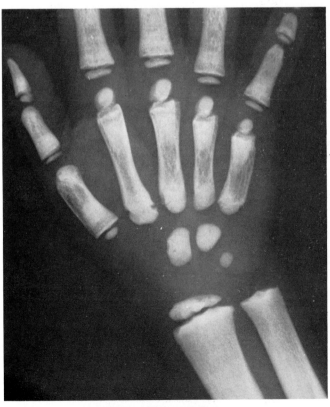

FIGURE 132   MASTER K.

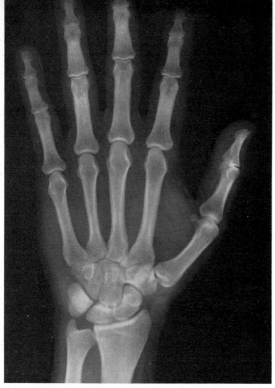

FIGURE 133   MRS. O.

This young lady, *Mrs. O*, cut her hand on some broken glass, and you request a radiograph to demonstrate any embedded foreign material.

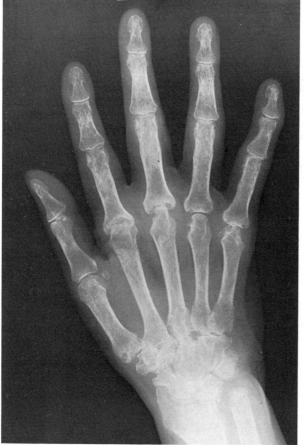

FIGURE 134   MISS S.

Miss S is a pleasant spinster schoolteacher who has been unable to work during the past eight years and now walks with great difficulty. She comes to you complaining of severe epigastric pains and one episode of "coffee-ground" vomitus.

This elderly lady, *Mrs. W*, has had intermittent pain in her hands and other joints for many years. Three weeks ago she fell and sprained her wrist. There was no fracture, but since then she has had throbbing pain in the wrist and hand, at times of unbearable intensity.

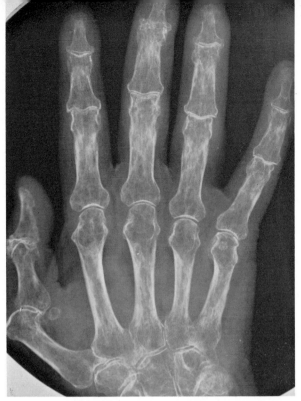

FIGURE 135   MRS. W.

Mr. L has had intermittent attacks of intense pain in his right hand and left foot for 20 years. His father and grandfather were similarly afflicted.

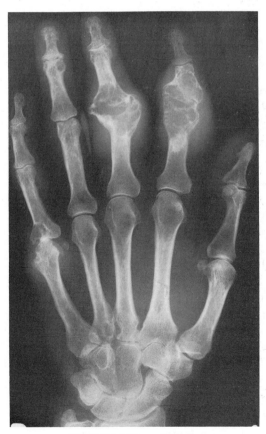

FIGURE 136   MR. L.

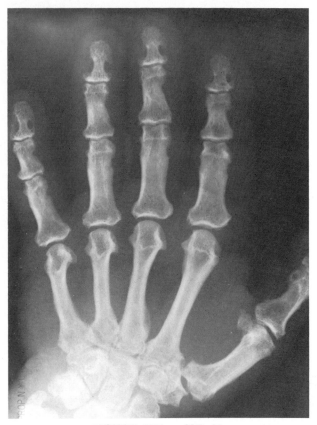

FIGURE 137   MR. N.

Mr. N is 32 years old and comes to you because last winter's hat and gloves, at that time a perfect fit, are now extremely small for him. His wife also has noted a great change in his facial appearance, particularly after comparison with last summer's snapshots.

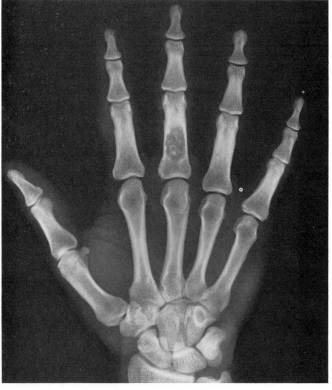

FIGURE 138   MR. D.

Mr. D caught his fingers in a car door. There is no external sign of injury when you examine him, but because he is complaining bitterly you request just this one view of the hand.

INSTRUCTIONS, QUESTIONS AND ACROSTIC

The game here is to find a patient to fit each of the roentgen descriptions below. Enter that patient's initial in the blank to the right. You may not actually use all the illustrations. Several patients are described more than once.

1. There is a patchy loss of spongiosa and cortical thinning in all the bones, consistent with severe osteoporosis. There is also marked narrowing and destruction of the distal interphalangeal joints. _____

2. The bones are generally too short but the mid-shaft diameter is normal. _____,_____

3. A disease of kings and other high livers. _____

4. There are three areas of localized soft-tissue swelling, with destruction of underlying bone. _____

5. There are irregular erosions of the heads of the metacarpals and also of the carpal bones. _____

6. There is a solitary, lytic, moderately rapidly growing tumor. _____

7. There is periarticular soft-tissue calcification. _____

8. There is generalized increase in density of all the bones. _____

9. There is a congenital defect of cartilage proliferation in growing bone. _____

10. A solitary lesion has expanded the cortex until it is only a thin shell, in places not visible. _____

11. There has been absorption of the tufts of all distal phalanges. _____

12. There is notable increase in soft-tissue thickness, generally. The bones are normal in length but increased in diameter. _____

13. A solitary, definitely benign lesion. _____

14. There is absence of the ulnar styloid process and involvement of metacarpo-phalangeal joints but little change about the interphalangeal joints. _____

ANSWERS

(Do not read until you have completed the exercise.)

Mrs. H has a rather agressive-looking solitary lesion; microscopically it proved to be a malignant giant-cell tumor. From its roentgen appearance, because it has eroded the cortex completely in places, one cannot be sure that it is benign. There may be a pathologic fracture present, although such fractures occur in bone weakened by either benign or malignant tumors. The precise diagnosis here would not be known until after the surgical excision and microscopic study, but the radiographic appearance would suggest that the lesion is malignant.

Master E is an achondroplastic dwarf.

Mr. A has a condition known as sclerodactyly, which is related to the collagen diseases — progressive systemic sclerosis (scleroderma), which this patient ultimately proved to have. There is often periarticular soft-tissue calcification.

Master K clearly has osteopetrosis. We have seen a case earlier in this volume. This one presents the interesting "bone within a bone" appearance seen in patients with this condition. It is thought to be due to transient amelioration of the inborn defect for a short time during active growth of the bone.

Mrs. O's hand film is, of course, normal. (Can glass be seen on radiographs?)

Miss S has advanced rheumatoid arthritis. The other cardinal features (in addition to those referred to in the acrostic) are juxta-articular osteoporosis and joint narrowing and destruction. The causes of osteoporosis in this disease are many. Acutely, it is usually juxta-articular and caused by increased vascularity about the inflamed joints. Later, with severe deformity, osteoporosis occurs because of disuse. Steroid therapy also results in generalized osteoporosis because of the catabolic effects of the hormone on bone. Could this also explain the history of gastrointestinal hemorrhage?

Mrs. W has degenerative joint disease of multiple small joints of the hands. There is thinning of joint cartilage and proliferative change (the addition of new bone, osteophytes, at the margins of the joints) – characteristically at the distal interphalangeal joints. This gives rise to the hard juxta-articular nodules known as Heberden's nodes. Mrs. W also has Sudeck's post-traumatic atrophy.

Mr. L is suffering from an inherited defect of purine metabolism, resulting in the clinical syndrome of gouty arthritis. The etiology of arthritis in gout is not entirely clear but seems to be related to the deposition of uric acid crystals in periarticular soft tissues. The typical changes of moderately advanced disease are seen here, with sharply gouged-out destructive lesions of juxta-articular bone. There is no tendency toward symmetry, as in rheumatoid arthritis. Note also that there is no apparent loss of articular cartilage as one would see in rheumatoid and degenerative arthritis.

Mr. N is suffering from the effects on adult bone of excessive secretion of pituitary growth hormone, probably by an eosinophilic adenoma of the pituitary. Because the epiphyses are fused, growth in length is not possible. Growth in diameter as the result of excessive periosteal bone deposition occurs. The soft tissues are also stimulated and become thicker in acromegaly. These patients have marked coarsening of facial features, with prominence of the eyebrows, forehead, and jaw. Note that over-production of bone has resulted in bridging between distal phalangeal tufts and shafts.

Mr. D has a small, benign enchondroma of his third proximal phalanx. It was found, as so many of them are, incidentally. They occasionally become large enough to make the bone prone to pathologic fracture. Note the characteristic calcification within the lesion.

NOW – – – – – –

WE'LL SHAKE HANDS!

INDEX

(NOTE: This is not really a formal index at all! Rather, it is simply meant to help you find something you want to see over again. Page numbers in **boldface** refer to page on which illustration may be found; those in lightface refer to discussion in the text.)